Advance praise for *Supporting Caregivers of Children with ADHD*

Chronis-Tuscano, O'Brien, and Danko present a clear, easy-to-follow manual "must-read" for therapists and educators working with parents of children with ADHD. The integration of "traditional" parent management procedures with emotion regulation strategies for parents is unique, representing a major advancement in the treatment of ADHD. I couldn't recommend this book more!

—**Rex Forehand**, PhD, University Distinguished Professor, University of Vermont

Timely, evidence-based, sensitive, accessible, flexible, and practical, *Supporting Caregivers of Children with ADHD* is an invaluable resource for working with parents of children with ADHD. Removing parent blame but not parent responsibility, it integrates behavioral and CBT strategies for parents who themselves have elements of ADHD, depression, emotion dysregulation, stress reactivity, and executive dysfunction. Highest recommendation!

—**Stephen P. Hinshaw**, PhD, UC Berkeley and UC San Francisco

Across the decades, experts in ADHD have created an array of effective parent training procedures that demonstrably improve child outcomes. This impressive book guides clinicians in the use of those well-established procedures, but it adds much more: strategies for personalizing treatment to fit the child and family, and a much-needed emphasis on support for the mental health and well-being of parents who are on the front lines of intervention. Parents who can manage their own emotions, cognitions, and responses to stress will be better equipped to provide what their children need; the book shows how parents can build those strengths. This innovative blend of venerable parent training procedures, novel personalizing strategies, and empirically guided support for parents makes this remarkable book a genuine tour de force.

—**John R. Weisz**, PhD, ABPP, Professor of Psychology, Harvard University

T0320780

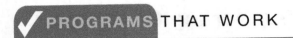

Supporting Caregivers of Children with ADHD

An Integrated Parenting Program

THERAPIST GUIDE

ANDREA CHRONIS-TUSCANO

KELLY O'BRIEN

CHRISTINA M. DANKO

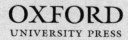

OXFORD
UNIVERSITY PRESS

OXFORD
UNIVERSITY PRESS

Oxford University Press is a department of the University of Oxford. It furthers
the University's objective of excellence in research, scholarship, and education
by publishing worldwide. Oxford is a registered trade mark of Oxford University
Press in the UK and certain other countries.

Published in the United States of America by Oxford University Press
198 Madison Avenue, New York, NY 10016, United States of America.

CIP data is on file at the Library of Congress
ISBN 978–0–19–094011–9

9 8 7 6 5 4 3 2 1

Printed by Marquis, Inc., Canada

This book is dedicated to the memories of my mother, grandmother, and brother Nick who illustrated for me the protective effects of warm, consistent parenting on child mental health. This book is also dedicated to Paul, Ravi and Gabe who remind me everyday how rewarding and challenging parenting can be. You also gave me a lot of great material for this book! My love for you is immeasurable.

—Andrea Chronis-Tuscano

For my biggest self-care supporters: Reece, our parents, and the self-care warriors. And for my biggest teachers: Ethen, Desmond, and Eliza.

—Kelly O'Brien

Dedicated with love to Sean, Michael, and Sarah.

—Christina M. Danko

Stunning developments in healthcare have taken place over the past several years, but many of our widely accepted interventions and strategies in mental health and behavioral medicine have been brought into question by research evidence as not only lacking benefit, but perhaps inducing harm (Barlow, 2010). Other strategies have been proved effective using the best current standards of evidence, resulting in broad-based recommendations to make these practices more available to the public (McHugh & Barlow, 2012). Several recent developments are behind this revolution. First, we have arrived at a much deeper understanding of pathology, both psychological and physical, which has led to the development of new, more precisely targeted interventions. Second, our research methodologies have improved substantially, such that we have reduced threats to internal and external validity, making the outcomes more directly applicable to clinical situations. Third, governments around the world and healthcare systems and policymakers have decided that the quality of care should improve, that it should be evidence-based, and that it is in the public's interest to ensure that this happens (Barlow, 2004; Institute of Medicine, 2001, 2015; Weisz & Kazdin, 2017).

Of course, the major stumbling block for clinicians everywhere is the accessibility of newly developed evidence-based psychological interventions. Workshops and books can go only so far in acquainting responsible and conscientious practitioners with the latest behavioral healthcare practices and their applicability to individual patients. This series, Programs ThatWork™, is devoted to communicating these exciting new interventions for children and adolescents to clinicians on the frontlines of practice.

The manuals and workbooks in this series contain step-by-step detailed procedures for assessing and treating specific problems and diagnoses. But this series also goes beyond the books and manuals by providing ancillary materials that will approximate the supervisory process in assisting practitioners in the implementation of these procedures in their practice.

In our emerging healthcare system, the growing consensus is that evidence-based practice offers the most responsible course of action for the mental health professional. All behavioral healthcare clinicians deeply desire to provide the best possible care for their patients. In this series, our aim is to close the dissemination and information gap and make that possible.

This therapist guide for the treatment of youth with attention-deficit/hyperactivity disorder (ADHD) and their parents is aimed at clinicians who have some familiarity with structured behavioral and cognitive-behavioral therapies (CBT) for children, adolescents, and adults. Modules integrate foundational behavioral principles involved in evidence-based parenting interventions (e.g., praise, contingency management, working with schools) with CBT skills used to treat executive functioning and internalizing problems in adults (e.g., adaptive thinking, relaxation, organizational skills). In addition, elements of emotion-focused treatments and mindfulness are incorporated throughout—all with the ultimate goal of teaching parents to effectively scaffold their children's behavioral and emotional regulation by creating a calm and consistent home environment. This intervention is based on a rigorous program of research demonstrating its effectiveness, and was designed and tested by a leading authority in the science of parenting interventions for ADHD and her colleagues.

Anne Marie Albano, Editor-in-Chief
David H. Barlow, Editor-in-Chief
Programs *That Work*

References

Barlow, D. H. (2004). Psychological treatments. *American Psychologist, 59,* 869–878.

Barlow, D. H. (2010). Negative effects from psychological treatments: A perspective. *American Psychologist, 65*(2), 13–20.

Institute of Medicine. (2001). *Crossing the quality chasm: A new health system for the 21st century.* Washington, DC: National Academy Press.

Institute of Medicine. (2015). *Psychosocial interventions for mental and substance use disorders: A framework for establishing evidence-based standards.* Washington, DC: National Academy Press.

McHugh, R. K., & Barlow, D. H. (2012). *Dissemination and implementation of evidence-based psychological interventions.* Oxford: Oxford University Press.

Weisz, J. R., & Kazdin, A. E. (2017). *Evidence-based psychotherapies for children and adolescents* (3rd ed.). New York: Guilford.

Contents

Acknowledgments

The ideas in this therapist guide began with Andrea Chronis-Tuscano's doctoral dissertation and have evolved in her laboratory at the University of Maryland, College Park, over almost two decades. Many people contributed to the evolution of this therapist guide, beginning with Stephanie A. Gamble, William E. Pelham, Jr., and John E. Roberts at the University at Buffalo. The input and insights of many former University of Maryland students/trainees and collaborators have been invaluable as this integrated treatment program was iteratively developed and refined over a period of many years, including (in alphabetical order): Tana Clarke, Yamalis Diaz, Heather A. Jones, Laura Knight, Erin Lewis-Morrarty, Heather Mazursky-Horowitz, Abigail Mintz-Romirowsky, Veronica Raggi, Mary Rooney, Karen Seymour, Jennifer Strickland, Sharon R. Thomas, Christine H. Wang, and many others. We were also fortunate to consult with Russell Barkley, Carl Lejuez, Peter Lewinsohn, Joan Luby, Jim Murphy, John Seeley, Charlotte Johnston, and Joel Sherrill with regard to the development and delivery of specific treatment components. Finally, the authors wish to thank the National Institutes of Health for their support to Dr. Chronis-Tuscano for related projects that facilitated the development of these ideas and evaluation of the various treatment components.

Introduction

In his recent book, *Getting Ahead of ADHD*, Dr. Joel Nigg describes how children with attention-deficit/hyperactivity disorder (ADHD) are more sensitive and reactive to their environments relative to their peers without ADHD (Nigg, 2017). Getting less sleep, having a cold, a disruption in routine, hearing mom and dad's argument—things that might easily "roll off the back" of a more even-tempered child often cause a great deal of upset for the child with ADHD who is prone to emotional dysregulation. Even positive events and emotions, like having out-of-town visitors or anticipating an upcoming family vacation or the last day of school before summer break, can throw off those children with ADHD who have difficulty regulating their positive as well as negative emotions.

Similarly, W. Thomas Boyce refers to children who are more sensitive to their environments in his book *The Orchid and the Dandelion* (Boyce, 2019). Many children are like dandelions; they will thrive and survive under a variety of conditions. Orchids, on the other hand, require a level of nurturance to reach their full potential. Under the right conditions, they will evolve into magnificent flowers, surpassing the beauty of dandelions. Thus, Boyce refers to orchids not so much in terms of their *vulnerability*, but more so in terms of their *sensitivity* to the environment and quality of care. The "orchid versus dandelion" is therefore a fitting metaphor for the protective nature of the parenting environment in enhancing the well-being and long-term success of children with ADHD.

Although it is well-established that the etiology (causes) of ADHD is largely genetic and neurobiological, ample longitudinal research evidence demonstrates that the quality of parenting and parent–child relationships can influence the extent to which youth with ADHD are impaired in their functioning (e.g., academically and socially) and how they fare over time (e.g., whether they develop co-occurring mood, behavioral, or substance use disorders). However, this is not a "one-way street": Children also greatly influence parent behaviors and well-being! In line with a developmental-transactional model of ADHD in families (Johnston & Chronis-Tuscano, 2015), parent and child characteristics each contribute to parent–child interactions and the parent–child relationship—and, ultimately, predict how the child with ADHD fares over time. (Refer to Figure I.1). In other words, the manner in which a parent responds to their child with ADHD can influence both the severity and course of the child's present and future difficulties. At the

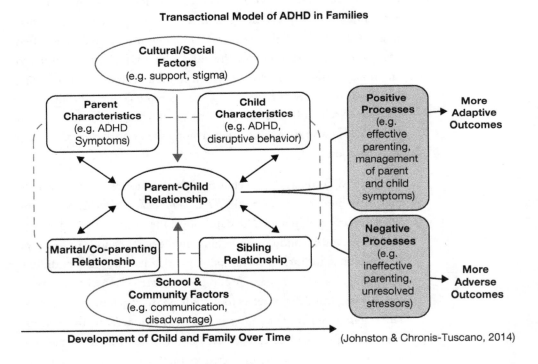

Figure I.1

Developmental-transactional model of attention-deficit/hyperactivity disorder (ADHD) within the family context.

Reproduced with permission from: Johnston, C., & Chronis-Tuscano, A. (2014). Families and ADHD. In R. A. Barkley (Ed.), *Attention-deficit hyperactivity disorder: A handbook for diagnosis and treatment, 4th ed.* (pp. 191–209). New York: Guilford.

same time, difficult child behavior often evokes harsh responses from caregivers, leading to increasing problems over time.

What makes this process even more challenging for many families is that ADHD, and many of the problems that go along with it—like executive functioning deficits, emotional dysregulation, and co-occurring depression—are highly heritable. For example, almost half of mothers of children with ADHD have a lifetime history of major depression and 25–50% of children with ADHD have parents with high levels of ADHD symptoms themselves (Johnston & Chronis-Tuscano, 2015). This means that some (if not many) parents of children with ADHD struggle with similar problems (even if not at diagnosable levels), making it much harder for many parents of children with ADHD to create the consistent, calm, and organized environment in which the child with ADHD is most likely to thrive. In other words, it is challenging for parents to scaffold the child with ADHD's learning and social environment if the parents themselves struggle with disorganization, inattention, poor planning, and other executive functioning difficulties. Similarly, it is challenging for a parent who frequently displays difficulties regulating their *own* emotions to *model* remaining calm in order to teach the child how to effectively manage their emotions. This is particularly important for children with ADHD who are at elevated risk for the development of depression by virtue of their difficulty regulating emotions (Seymour et al., 2012; Seymour, Chronis-Tuscano, Iwamoto, Kurdziel, & MacPherson, 2014).

What's more, the evidence-based behavioral parenting techniques that are the cornerstone of our very best therapies for children with ADHD, oppositional defiant disorder (ODD), conduct disorder (CD), and externalizing problems more broadly take an awful lot of motivation, effort, and energy—much more than a parent who is feeling extremely stressed, depressed, or depleted can give. Even parents with the very best intentions may not have the self-regulation skills, motivation, or organization to do what our evidence-based behavioral interventions require.

Given all of this, you may be asking: "What can therapists do to help?" Unfortunately, most of our evidence-based treatment approaches focus on behavioral parenting techniques and organizational skills that help children with ADHD be successful, but such skills and techniques often are quite challenging for many parents to implement given their own difficulties. Until now, few intervention programs for children with ADHD have given adequate attention to this very important issue, and none has integrated the focus on parent mental health with parenting in exactly the way we do in this program.

Transactional Model of ADHD in Families

It is widely accepted that the causes of ADHD lie in the brain. ADHD is highly genetic—it is actually more genetically transmitted than height and IQ! More specifically, studies have shown that the heritability of ADHD is 70–80% throughout the lifespan (Franke et al., 2012), and ample research shows that the structure and function of the brains of individuals with ADHD differ from those of individuals without ADHD (Faraone et al., 2005). However, a large and growing body of research also shows that the *environment* can influence the extent to which ADHD is impairing the child's functioning at any given time. In particular, the quality of the *social* environment—including most prominently the family and parenting (but also a child's relationships and interactions with teachers and peers)—is associated with the degree of functional impairment experienced by the child and the extent to which ADHD-related problems evolve into other more serious comorbid conditions that can lead to devastating outcomes.

Depression, anxiety, suicide, and substance use in adolescence and adulthood occur at far higher rates in individuals diagnosed with ADHD in childhood, and some research has shown that parenting can exacerbate or mitigate these negative outcomes. For example, research by Brooke Molina and colleagues demonstrated that parenting moderated the association between childhood ADHD and adolescent problematic alcohol use. Specifically, childhood ADHD predicted alcohol use frequency at age 17 *only when* parental knowledge of the teen's friendships, activities, and whereabouts was below median levels for the sample (Molina et al., 2012). Similarly, our prior work demonstrated that early positive parenting (observed when the children were 4–6 years old) predicted the course of conduct problems in children with ADHD when controlling for baseline child conduct problems, parent psychopathology, and other potentially confounding factors. In other words, some environments can effectively scaffold the academic, social, and emotional functioning of children with ADHD so that they are resilient to developmental risks commonly associated with ADHD. In other cases, for a variety of reasons that may exceed the parents' control (e.g., in the context of severe economic deprivation), parent factors may exert less influence (Miller, Gustafsson, et al., 2018).

Of course, interactions between the child with ADHD and their social world are complex and transactional (Johnston & Chronis-Tuscano, 2015; Figure I.1 illustrates the model). Children with ADHD are not always easy to be around! Many are loud, reactive, full of energy, and do not tend to honor physical boundaries. They may take longer and require more hands-on supervision to complete everyday morning, homework, and bedtime routines due to their distractibility and difficulty breaking down and following through on multistep tasks. As children get older, parents and teachers increasingly expect them to complete these tasks more independently and have less patience for the level of supervision and support they require. Indeed, youth with ADHD continue to require a developmentally *in*appropriate level of parental support throughout adolescence and young adulthood.

Frustrated by this, parents may sometimes react by yelling or spanking, which can contribute to a negative spiral and poor parent–child relations. This further feeds into negative thoughts-feelings-emotions for both the child and parent.

In line with this transactional model, the very same parent might look quite different with a child who is temperamentally easier, so in this way the more challenging child is truly *evoking* parenting responses that further contribute to negative developmental outcomes. In other words, it is easy to stay positive and connected to a well-behaved or easygoing child, but it is much more challenging to respond calmly and consistently to a child with behavioral challenges. Similarly, a temperamentally easier child may do well regardless of the quality of parenting (a "dandelion"), but children with ADHD require parents to be even more organized and on top of things in order to succeed (they are "orchids").

Somehow, despite this natural pull to respond negatively to difficult child behavior, some parents still manage to remain calm (at least most of the time!) and maintain a positive, warm, and emotionally close relationship with their child with ADHD. Some of our research has shown that certain parents are at greater risk for responding to child misbehavior with negative or critical parenting behaviors by virtue of their own genetics (Lee et al., 2008). But interestingly, in this study, negative parenting behavior *was only apparent* when children displayed more challenging behavior during the interaction, again supporting this transactional model whereby child misbehavior evokes negative parenting responses among parents who are themselves at risk for behaving this way (e.g., as a result of their own genetic makeup) (Lee et al., 2008).

Our research has also shown that mothers of children with ADHD who have their own executive functioning deficits (i.e., on working memory and planning tasks) engage in less scaffolding with their school-aged children (Mazursky-Horowitz et al., 2018). Additionally, we have found that mothers' emotion regulation difficulties interact with child ADHD symptoms to predict harsh parenting and the child's development of emotion regulation (Oddo et al., in press). And maternal emotion dysregulation and child ADHD interact to predict the trajectory of depressive symptoms across adolescence (Oddo et al., 2019). Thus, it is not only mothers with a diagnosis of depression or ADHD who demonstrate difficulties with parenting, but the full range of maternal difficulties with executive functioning and emotion regulation also is associated with less adaptive parenting, especially when the child demonstrates ADHD symptoms. These processes can have serious consequences for the long-term outcomes of youth with ADHD.

What we know very clearly from the research is that warm, supportive parenting is *extraordinarily* protective for children with ADHD, whereas negative verbal and physical parental behavior exacerbates risk for additional emotional and behavioral difficulties as children with ADHD move through development (e.g., Chronis et al., 2007; Harold et al., 2013).

So how do we break this cycle? How do we help parents who struggle with being warm and consistent and structured despite their children's difficulties? Parenting a child with ADHD requires specialized parenting. Parents are instructed to provide a therapeutic environment for their child, and the demands are high: to be *pro*active (rather than *re*active), stay consistent, and manage the parent's own frustration in emotionally charged situations so that they can be effective. This is easier said than done, particularly when parents themselves are presenting with depressive or anxious symptoms, ADHD, or high levels of environmental stress. We can validate these challenges and instill hope by providing parents with cognitive-behavioral therapy (CBT) strategies that can assist them with providing a therapeutic environment for their child. We can also give parents permission, through psychoeducation and skill building, to be kind to themselves. In other words, yelling now and then (while not ideal) does not erase their hard work and generally supportive approach to their children. Everyone makes mistakes sometimes, but the goal is to take a general approach that is typically calm, consistent, and not chaotic!

Parenting Interventions Involving a Focus on Parent Mental Health

Behavioral parent training (BPT) research began with pioneers like Constance Hanf, who developed the two-stage "child's play," "parent's play," parent training model (Reitman & McMahon, 2013). Hanf's work inspired many behavioral parent management training programs, including those developed by Russell Barkley, Sheila Eyberg, Rex Forehand, Alan Kazdin, Bob McMahon, Gerald Patterson, Matt Sanders, Robert Wahler, Carolyn Webster-Stratton, and others. BPT programs have been backed by more than 40 years of sound empirical research and are considered a well-established treatment for ADHD and oppositional behavior in children and, to a lesser extent, adolescents (Evans, Owens, Wymbs, & Ray, 2018).

Over the years, some of these parenting researchers have attempted to include enhanced versions of parent training with modules focused on parent mental health, typically taking a cognitive-behavioral approach (Griest et al., 1982; Sanders, Markie-Dadds, Tully, & Bor, 2000; Sanders & McFarland, 2000; Webster-Stratton, 1990). In line with this work, our program of research has focused on several aspects of parent mental health that can make parenting more challenging, including maternal depression, parental ADHD, executive functioning, stress reactivity, and emotion regulation (e.g., Chronis et al., 2007; Chronis-Tuscano et al., 2008; Mazursky-Horowitz et al., 2015). Not surprisingly, these parent characteristics contribute to parenting difficulties and youth outcomes both cross-sectionally and over time for children and adolescents with ADHD (see Johnston & Chronis-Tuscano, 2015, for a review). And we have examined various ways to target these parent emotional, behavioral, and executive functioning difficulties as part of a comprehensive and integrative approach to the treatment of children with ADHD within the family context, in line with our transactional model (refer to Figure I.1). We, and others, have conducted well-controlled studies showing that *integrating* and *infusing* content targeting parents' own thoughts, feelings, behaviors, and emotion coaching throughout a parent training program add incremental value beyond standard parent training on outcomes including parent well-being, parenting quality, and child outcomes (e.g., Chronis-Tuscano et al., 2013).

Foundational Theories/Models for This Treatment Program

ABCs of Child Behavior

Most evidence-based behavioral interventions have as their cornerstone a "functional analysis" of behavior to examine environmental factors that make it more or less likely that a desired or undesirable behavior will occur (**A = Antecedents**). Antecedents may include people, settings, time of day, level of structure, and demands that make it more or less likely that a child will behave in a certain way (either positively or negatively). For example, during our assessments when reviewing the child's developmental history, we often hear from parents that a child was successful in second grade when the teacher was calm, highly structured, positive, and/or seated the child at the front of the class. In contrast, first and third grades were disastrous when a teacher was less structured, reactive, or critical. These types of examples provided by parents can help to illustrate how different classroom contexts can yield quite different child behaviors and different levels of adaptation. Our goal, of course, is to help parents to create a context that will support their child's positive development by encouraging appropriate behavior.

Consequences (C) refer to what occurs immediately *after* the child's behavior that makes it more or less likely that the behavior will occur again in the future. Following from the principles of operant conditioning, an individual will be more likely to repeat a behavior that is followed by a reinforcer and less likely to repeat a behavior that is followed by a punishment (Skinner, 1963). Examples of common consequences include praise, adult attention, peer attention, yelling, spanking, time out, or loss of a privilege. Of course, parents (and teachers) often inadvertently reinforce misbehavior by paying too much attention to child misbehavior, often ignoring a child's efforts or successes. Even negative attention from parents, teachers, and peers can be reinforcing for children.

Over time, some parents and teachers may fail to notice when a child is behaving appropriately, take a "let sleeping dogs lie" attitude, or they may fundamentally not agree with praising children for behavior that they "should" be doing in the first place. Focusing almost exclusively on a child's *misbehavior* can have a detrimental effect on the parent–child relationship and damage the child's self-esteem.

The strategies laid out in this program involve encouraging parents to give their attention to appropriate behaviors and minimize attention to misbehavior except when those behaviors are dangerous and require negative, nonphysical consequences. This approach is often referred to as "differential attention." Several of the modules in our guide address positive (e.g., labeled praise) and negative consequences (e.g., active ignoring, time out) to promote positive and reduce negative behaviors.

Another challenge in this operant model is that consequences need to be *immediate* and *consistent* to change behavior. Within our transactional model, this can be challenging based on both parent and child characteristics. We know that "reinforcement sensitivity" has been proposed as an important factor within ADHD (Castellanos & Tannock, 2002; Luman, Tripp, & Scheres, 2010; Nigg & Casey, 2005; Sonuga-Barke, 2002). In other words, children with ADHD are more sensitive to rewards compared to children without ADHD (which is good), but require those rewards to be more *immediate, frequent,* and *consistent* in order to be effective in changing their behavior.

Now, from the parent perspective, considering that parents of children with ADHD often have similar difficulties with executive functioning (e.g., persistence on a task, organization, sustained attention, emotion regulation) and are also at increased risk for mood disorders (characterized by low motivation, fatigue, negativity), it can be extremely demanding for many parents of children with ADHD to consistently keep up with this high level of structure and frequent consequences. To address this difficulty, in this program, we have integrated evidence-based cognitive-behavioral techniques to directly address these parental difficulties within the parenting context.

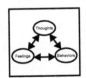

Cognitive-Behavioral Model

Thoughts

A cognitive-behavioral perspective highlights the bidirectional interplay between thoughts, feelings, and behaviors (Beck, 1979; Ellis & Grieger, 1986). In other words, thoughts, feelings, and behaviors each influence one another in a dynamic and reciprocal manner. CBT is considered an evidence-based treatment for adults with depression, anxiety, ADHD, and many other problems frequently experienced by parents of children with ADHD (Chronis et al., 2003). In CBT, the client is taught skills that target maladaptive thoughts, feelings, and behaviors.

We have found in our clinical work and research that this model indeed fits quite well when working with parents of children with ADHD and related disorders. Parents with whom we work often express unhelpful thoughts, like: "Things are never going to change," "Maybe this is all my fault," "She is doing this to me on purpose," "He is just lazy," "He will never change," "She will never amount to anything," "I am not a very good parent," "I don't enjoy being with my child at all anymore," "None of these strategies (e.g., time out) work for my child." Negative thoughts about oneself, one's child, or the potential efficacy of the behavioral therapy can greatly undermine your work with families of children with ADHD and pose a barrier to optimal treatment response. In this program, we will directly intervene with these thoughts.

Psychoeducation can be a helpful first step in terms of challenging some of the negative thinking parents have in relation to their children with ADHD. Understanding that there are indeed differences between the structure and function of brains of children with and without ADHD can help to dispel the myth that their children are doing some of these annoying things on purpose.

> **Therapist Note**
>
> ADHD behaviors are rarely purposeful, but even for children with ODD it is helpful to consider that children do better when they can.

Learning that many children with ADHD have executive functioning deficits can help parents to understand and empathize with the child's difficulty in staying on task and completing multistep tasks/routines independently. And the knowledge that emotion dysregulation is now considered a third component of ADHD can help parents to better understand that some of their children's intense emotional reactions to seemingly minor things are also a part of this brain-based condition.

Balancing the brain and genetic basis of ADHD with the need for the child to, at the same time, be accountable for their actions is sometimes challenging. In other words, we indeed want to support parents in calmly implementing clear and consistent expectations and consequences (making the child accountable for their actions) despite the fact that the child is not purposely behaving this way. Reframing child behavior in this way can help to reduce parent anger and frustration and help parents take a more sensitive and empathic view of their children.

In this program, it is exceedingly important to convey the message to parents that their child's difficulties are *not* the parents' fault. This is a common thought expressed by parents with ADHD. In other words, we, as therapists, need to praise parents as much as possible and to send the message that, while the child's problems are not the parents' fault, with your support parents can learn to structure the home environment in a manner that will help the child to be successful, both now and in the future. Note that this dichotomy can be difficult for many parents to grasp. If it is not their fault, then why are we focusing so much of the therapy on them? Why, if this is a brain-based condition, isn't medication enough? This is where the therapist's knowledge of the literature comes in, showing that combined treatments best address the impairments associated with ADHD (Jensen et al., 2001) and that parenting quality predicts the trajectory of ADHD symptoms (Harold et al., 2013) and development of comorbidities (Chronis et al., 2007).

Finally, throughout this program, it is important to *instill hope* in parents that their child's behavior, parental reactions to the child, and the overall family situation can change with your support. Unlike other treatment programs, here we will be paying attention to the parent's well-being in addition to their parenting and their child's behavior, to enhance parents' ability to do their very best with their child. As the saying goes, "You cannot pour from an empty cup!"

Feelings

Sometimes parents of children with ADHD have difficulty managing their own emotions, as we have described. This difficulty may have preceded the child's difficulties, or sometimes the child's difficulties may contribute to or exacerbate the parents' feelings of emotional upset. Or, there may be shared biological underpinnings for this pattern that were passed from parents to the child. Most often, it is some combination.

However, to be most effective at delivering the behavioral parenting components and to stay even-keeled in the face of difficult child behavior, we work with parents to develop skills to remain calm in the face of stress. We work with parents to be *pro*active in their approach to parenting their child with ADHD, rather than emotionally *re*active. The ability to regulate one's feelings can also increase a parent's effectiveness at working collaboratively with their child's school, not to mention with the co-parent and in the workplace. After all, the ability to effectively manage stress impacts most areas of our lives.

For this reason, this therapist guide includes several modules (or sections of modules) aimed at directly impacting one's feelings in the moment, particularly learning and implementing relaxation and mindfulness skills. However, many of the other modules indirectly intend to impact parents' feelings of stress and low mood via behavioral changes. For example, if a parent prioritizes taking time to exercise daily or getting 7–8 hours of sleep per night, they will be less prone to experiencing negative emotions (Pemberton & Tyszkiewicz, 2016).

Behaviors

Despite the importance of changing thoughts and feelings, the easiest target (or "lowest hanging fruit") within a CBT model is behavior, which often leads to corresponding changes in thoughts and feelings. For this reason, we start by working with parents on changing behaviors related to their own self-care (and, of course, their parenting). Parents, in general, tend to neglect their own needs in the service of their children. This may be true even more so when their children have special needs. However, we argue in this program that parents of demanding children have an even *greater* need to take time for themselves.

A major theme of this program is that parents are in a much better place to parent their difficult child when they have had an opportunity to "recharge." Peter Lewinsohn's research suggests that, in general, positive social interactions and activities that help us to feel competent have the most profound impact on our mood (Lewinsohn, Munoz, Youngren, & Zeiss, 1986). We all differ in terms of what specific activities help us to feel good, but, in general, adequate sleep, exercise, fresh air, and pleasurable social interactions have a powerful influence on our mood.

Trying to fit in these pleasant activities is not always easy for parents, but we begin with "baby steps," with the intention of making self-care a priority for parents and their parenting. Before long, parents will notice the positive impact that even simple self-care activities have on their parenting and on their interactions with their children. This can, in turn, influence parent thoughts about the importance of taking time for themselves (consistent with our thoughts-feelings-behaviors framework). Rather than seeing self-care activities as a lower priority and even somewhat selfish, we try to help parents become aware of the positive ripple effects that prioritizing self-care can have on their family interactions.

For Whom Is This Program Appropriate?

This treatment program is intended for parents of 4- to 12-year-old children with ADHD who struggle with managing their own thoughts, emotions, and behaviors in a manner that interferes with effective parenting. The majority of our research on these integrated treatment components (CBT, emotion coaching) was conducted with depressed mothers or mothers with ADHD (Chronis-Tuscano et al., 2013, 2016). However, it is not just parents with *clinical levels* of depression, ADHD, or anger management problems who need extra support in creating an ideal environment for their child with ADHD: stress/mood regulation, energy level, and organizational skills fall on a continuum. Said differently, some of us are more organized, have more energy and motivation, are better planners, or are calmer and more flexible than others. Some parents struggle with their own health problems (e.g., insomnia, migraines, chronic illness), which may further contribute to the fatigue of parenting a difficult child. We would be remiss to suggest that parents struggling in any of these areas would not benefit from the treatment components focusing on parent well-being. Most parents would!

Theoretically, the skills and techniques contained within this guide can also be applied to families of children with *a range of emotional and behavioral difficulties*, including children with subthreshold ADHD or with disruptive behavior problems like noncompliance, anger, and difficult temperaments more characteristic of ODD or CD. Similarly, the principles of parent self-care and BPT discussed in this therapist guide could be applied to parents of children with internalizing problems.

In fact, one could argue that *all* parents could benefit from the skills put forth in this guide, regardless of their or their child's diagnostic status. That is why we take a *flexible* approach to the delivery of these modules, individualizing the amount of time spent on content to match the family's presenting problems and challenges.

Similarities and Differences with Other Treatment Programs

This program has similarities and differences with other interventions you may have used in the past. Like others, this program reviews basic behavioral principles that can help children with ADHD and related problems to be successful, such as adjusting the antecedents and consequences of a child's behavior to set the child up for success and reward positive behaviors, while at the same time using nonphysical discipline to punish more serious misbehaviors. These behavioral principles have been described in the writings of Hanf, Patterson,

Forehand, Eyberg, Webster-Stratton, Barkley, Sanders, Kazdin, and others for decades.

This program also involves the application of evidence-based CBT principles to adults: the parents. These principles are drawn from the Coping with Depression Course developed by Peter Lewinsohn (Lewinsohn et al., 1986) and the groundbreaking work of Aaron Beck and Albert Ellis with regard to cognitive therapy/restructuring (Beck, 1987; Ellis & Grieger, 1986).

The work of John Gottman and Lynn Fainsilber-Katz at the University of Washington on parent emotion coaching has also greatly influenced our thinking about parents as emotion coping models and coaches (Gottman & Declaire, 1998). Their longitudinal research has established the role of parent emotion coaching in children's development of emotion regulation. Until recently, emotion coaching has not been included in evidence-based BPT programs. However, several recent efforts to integrate emotion coaching with operant programs have yielded promising results for children with ADHD (e.g., Chronis-Tuscano et al., 2016; Herbert, Harvey, Roberts, Wichowski, & Lugo-Candelas, 2013) and preschoolers with depression (Luby, Barch, Whalen, Tillman, & Freedland, 2018).

Parent emotion coaching may be a particularly important treatment component for youth with ADHD because emotion regulation difficulties are now recognized as a third core feature of ADHD (along with inattention and hyperactivity/impulsivity). Moreover, a growing body of research demonstrates that emotion regulation mediates the association between ADHD and later depression (e.g., Seymour et al., 2012, 2014). This research suggests that the manner in which parents respond to their children's expressions of emotions can help or hinder the child or adolescent's development of emotion identification and regulation, which can have downstream effects on their emotional well-being (Oddo et al., in press).

What makes our program unique is that it *integrates* parent self-care (derived from CBT) with the behavioral parenting principles that are considered an evidence-based treatment for children with ADHD and disruptive behaviors. In other words, we apply CBT for parents *in the context of* parenting a child with ADHD. Other parent training manuals may instruct a parent to deliver commands in a neutral tone or to ignore minor misbehaviors, but they do not teach parents *how* to stay calm. Other efforts to provide enhancements to standard BPT to address parent mental health usually follow a standard course of parent training (Griest et al., 1982; Sanders, Markie-Dadds, Tully, & Bor, 2000; Sanders & McFarland, 2000; Webster-Stratton, 1990), rather than infusing or integrating a focus on parent mental health throughout the manual.

In our work, we have sometimes encountered questions about why we would not just refer a parent out for individual treatment. These questioners have suggested that we may be confusing the identified client. However, we feel strongly that an *integrative* approach is optimal given the bidirectional effects of child and parent mental health, in line with our transactional model of ADHD in families (Johnston & Chronis-Tuscano, 2015).

Importance of Maintaining a Supportive and Nonjudgmental Stance

For years, parents were blamed for biologically-based children's mental health concerns (e.g., autism, schizophrenia, and ADHD), and it is important to point out that this is not at all what we are trying to do in this book. Rather, we want to take a *supportive stance* with parents, helping them to acknowledge what is challenging for them (as well as their strengths) and supporting them with the skills they need to help their children be successful now and in the long term.

Parents of children with ADHD are truly asked to be "super parents." Sadly, however, when we expect some parents to consistently implement complex behavior management plans or homework plans and they cannot deliver, they are often left feeling inadequate and a failure; what's worse, some of these parents feel like they caused the child's problems to begin with. That is why it is crucial to introduce the skills and the theoretical model in an empathic and supportive manner that recognizes the parent, too, as a client who may have the best intentions—and really want to do their best for their child—but who may need skills and extra support to be able to provide that optimal environment.

Group Versus Individual Format

In our research, we tested some elements of this program in group format (Chronis-Tuscano et al., 2013) and other elements in individual format (e.g., Chronis-Tuscano et al., 2016). In practice, you can deliver this program in group or individual format, depending on what is most fitting in your setting. Both formats have obvious advantages. Groups provide social support for other parents "in the same boat" and can be cost efficient, but group programs are logistically challenging in many practice settings. For example, it can be difficult to find a time that works for everyone and to assemble a group of parents who are ready to begin treatment at the same time without making parents wait too long for treatment to begin (which can result in decreased motivation). Groups also make it difficult to personalize treatment to the unique needs of a particular parent, child, or family.

On the other hand, delivering this treatment in group (when feasible) is often helpful in dispelling some of the self-blame that certain parents are prone to. In other words, meeting other parents who are obviously very invested in and dedicated to their children's well-being and are similarly struggling can be helpful in normalizing a parent's experience. Hearing other parents say that they sometimes blame themselves when it is very obvious how much they invest in their children can help other parents to understand that they are not to blame either. It can be easier and more comfortable for parents to challenge another group member's negative thinking before they can challenge their own.

Additionally, the group format allows parents to showcase what has worked for them in the past. Often, some group members will have been successful with certain skills while struggling immensely with others; other group members may have opposite strengths and difficulties. This can contribute to a sense of parenting competence among participants, which can be lacking in many parents of children with ADHD. Finally, creating a community where group members can understand and help one another may combat some of the feelings of isolation that may arise for parents of children with ADHD.

Despite the many strengths of a group format, most practitioners find an individual format more feasible with their clients. For this reason, we set as default an individual format in this guide, which also assumes that the child is not present for sessions. We provide suggestions for the group format throughout each module to allow for flexibility in delivery.

Relevance of Modules/Content to Individual Families

Not all of the skills presented in the guide will be as relevant to every family with whom you work. You may therefore wish to emphasize (i.e., spend more time on) those modules that are most relevant to the concerns of a particular family. Some modules will be critical for all families (e.g., the foundational theories presented in Module 1), but there are other goals that may be more relevant for some parents than others (e.g., daily schedule, social skills, assertiveness). Similarly, some families may have already received a standard course of parent training and would therefore be familiar with special time, praise, and other behavior management skills. For these families, you may be able to spend relatively less time on those core behavioral parenting skills and relatively more time on the parent thoughts, feelings, and behaviors that can interfere with or facilitate consistent, effective use of these behavior management skills.

No two parents and children are alike, and treatments that are individualized to a family's needs are likely better received. For instance, the parent of a child who is predominantly inattentive and disorganized may be turned off by too much focus on how to respond to aggressive or defiant child behavior because it will not be viewed as salient and may lead to the parent feeling that this program is not right for them or their family. Focusing relatively greater emphasis on how to swiftly get through the morning or bedtime routine is going to be more salient for these families and will help to keep them engaged. Similarly, some parents are highly organized and/or socially skillful. Spending too much time on these aspects of a module viewed as less relevant may seem to parents like a waste of precious therapy time and resources.

You may wish to skip modules or goals that are less relevant to a particular family. Although this is tempting, we believe that most parents can learn helpful tips by touching on all of the modules in this book at least briefly, but the content can be covered more quickly for parents who are not struggling in a particular domain (e.g., scheduling or social skills). However, keep in mind that it is often not until you raise a particular topic that you learn something new about a parent (e.g., that they behave aggressively toward school staff or the co-parent, or use alcohol/substances to cope with stress), so don't *assume* that something is not a problem for a parent until you ask and have had an opportunity to discuss it.

Importance of Between-Session Practice

As in all behavioral and CBT programs, between-session practice of parenting and self-care skills is essential here. We avoid calling this practice "homework" (since some parents have had previous negative experiences with homework) and instead emphasize that we are trying to adjust elements of the home structure and parenting in a consistent way that eventually becomes automatic. You can use the analogy of learning to play a musical instrument. If you do not practice between weekly lessons with your piano teacher, you will not learn to play very well. Any time we are learning something new or changing a behavior, *repeated practice is essential.*

To highlight the importance of between-session practice and troubleshoot any issues that arise with the practice, as the therapist, it is critical to routinely review home practice. Spend at least 5–10 minutes at the beginning of each session on reviewing how home practice is going. However, unlike some other manuals, there is flexibility built in for those parents who need more time or therapist support to master a particular skill.

If the parent does not practice the skill or this is a particularly tough skill for the parent to implement, the CBT (thoughts-feelings-behaviors) model may be helpful in understanding *why* the parent did not practice. Is it an issue of the parent not fully buying in to the importance of the skill? Have they already decided that this approach will not work with their child? Is the suggested skill incongruent with the way the parent was raised or with the parent's culture? Does the parent anticipate push-back from the co-parent and/or other family members involved in child rearing? Did the parent simply forget to practice? Are there other practical issues standing in the way? It is critical to explore this and do a functional analysis of homework nonadherence to move forward with the program.

Parents with Low Motivation for Change

Some parents enter therapy for their child not expecting that a large amount of time will be spent working directly with them to change their behavior. They may be expecting what others have referred to as a "Jiffy Lube" approach—you drop your child off with the therapist while you sit in the waiting room reading a magazine (e.g., see Weisz, 2004). These parents will be very surprised to learn the relative emphasis and time that you (as the therapist) will spend with them in this program.

Every once in a while, you will encounter a parent who is less motivated for change. For this reason, some research groups have examined the addition of motivational interviewing (MI) to BPT (e.g., Nock & Kazdin, 2005; Scott & Dadds, 2009; Ingoldsby, 2010).

The overarching goal of MI is to strengthen one's "*motivation* for and *commitment* to a specific goal by eliciting and exploring the person's own reasons for change within an atmosphere of acceptance and compassion" (Miller & Rollnick, 2012, p. 29). By asking open-ended questions about reasons for help-seeking and the current family/parenting situation, you can *listen* intently for any "change talk"; that is, the parent vocalizing a desire for their own parenting reactions or behavior to be different in the future. You can then selectively *reflect* these statements back (e.g., "You really feel like something has to change"). People are far more likely to be persuaded based on their own words as compared to being told directly by a therapist (taking more of the "expert role") that they need to make a change.

Some open-ended questions that may evoke change talk include:

- *In what ways does this behavior concern you?*

- *How would you like things to be different, either in your own life or with your parenting or with your child?*
- *How would things be better if you learned to change your responses to your child?*
- *How would things be better if you prioritized your own well-being?*
- *What's your next step?*

Other aspects of MI include *expressing empathy* and *supporting self-efficacy*. As noted in other sections of this guide, parenting a child with ADHD can be really challenging, and no parent is going to respond in an optimal manner every time. Endeavor to instill hope and confidence that the parents you work with *can* make changes by focusing on their own mental health or self-care together with their implementation of evidence-based parenting skills.

 For additional resources that will help you to incorporate MI into your delivery of this program, we recommend the classic text by Miller and Rollnick (2012), which can be ordered with helpful training videos.

Who Is the Identified Client?

Some providers get caught up in defining "the identified client" when we suggest integrating a focus on the child/parenting with a parent's own mental health. They might suggest that the parent be referred out for therapy. Within a developmental-transactional framework, we argue that the two are so intertwined that this type of distinction is not as helpful as *focusing on the system* (with some exceptions; see later discussion). In other words, if the parent is struggling with their own emotion regulation or executive functioning (e.g., organizational) issues, these difficulties will most often be a huge obstacle in terms of creating the type of parenting environment that children with ADHD tend to thrive in. Ignoring the parents' own struggles will not help the parenting work and instead acts as a "brick wall" to making lasting changes in parenting and family functioning.

This treatment program involves an integration of behavioral parenting and parent-focused CBT skills in a way that separate treatment for the parent and child cannot fully achieve. Specifically, in this guide, we discuss how the parents' own difficulties play out in scenarios with their children, which can make the implementation of behavioral parenting strategies harder. By *explicitly* applying these CBT skills within the context of parenting, our intention is to improve the mental health of the child and parent, enhance their positive interactions, and ultimately improve the child's developmental outcomes (refer back to Figure I.1).

Referral of Parents for Individual and/or Couples Treatment

At the same time, therapists should stay attuned to more serious or pervasive parent difficulties that may warrant referral for individual, couples, or pharmacological treatment. For example, 25–50% of parents of children with ADHD have ADHD themselves (Johnston, Mash, Miller, & Ninowski, 2012). If, at any time, you suspect a parent has ADHD and that the skills included in this program are insufficient to address parent ADHD-related impairments, you may gently suggest that the parent consider obtaining an adult ADHD evaluation (and perhaps subsequently consider stimulant medication). Also, if the parent is experiencing occupational difficulty or serious problems in relationships beyond the parent–child dyad, you may recommend individual and/or couples therapy.

This is obviously a sensitive topic, but, to the extent that these problems are causing issues for the parent, they may directly or indirectly be affecting the child as well (via parent distress or interparental conflict). Just be careful (as always) about how you convey this message to avoid parent blaming/shaming, especially for parents who might be prone to such self-blaming thoughts and feelings.

Using the Therapist Guide

At the beginning of each module, you will find an overview of the goals for the module. The typical structure of each module is to review the home practice from the previous module, cover the new material, and then assign home practice based on the new material discussed. To facilitate covering the material from this therapist guide in session, we have included a brief therapist outline for each module in Appendix B at the end of this book. You can refer to this outline in session as a kind of "cheat sheet" or "Cliffs Notes" until you become more familiarized with the program. In addition, you might find it helpful to return to the introduction for reference as needed throughout treatment.

Summary

- The etiology of ADHD is largely genetic and neurobiological; however, the quality of parenting and parent–child relationships can influence the developmental trajectory of children with ADHD.
- There are higher rates of mental health disorders among parents of children with ADHD, and the associated impairments create challenges when implementing interventions for ADHD.
- For these and other reasons detailed in the introduction, this therapist guide was created to uniquely integrate a focus on parent mental health within a behavioral parenting intervention.
- The transactional model of ADHD describes the complex interactions between the child with ADHD and their social context.
- The ABC model is incorporated throughout this guide. Parents learn how to change antecedents and consequences to create an environmental context that will support their child's positive development.
- The cognitive-behavioral model is used throughout this guide to help parents modify their own thoughts, feelings, and behaviors to improve their mood and parenting.
- This program is designed for parents of children with ADHD who struggle with managing their own thoughts, emotions, and behaviors.
- It is important to take a supportive and nonjudgmental stance with parents and to not engage in parent blaming when delivering treatment content.
- There is flexibility in delivering the treatment in a group or individual format. Although the therapist guide is written for delivery to individual parents, suggestions for group delivery are incorporated throughout.
- There is also flexibility in the delivery of the modules. You may want to omit or go through some modules more quickly if parents need less support in certain areas (e.g., time management) or change the

order depending on other factors (e.g., deliver the school-focused sessions during the academic year).

- For the program to be successful, parents need to complete the between-session practice. Some parents may require additional support as well as help in problem-solving barriers to make this happen.
- MI is a valuable tool that can be incorporated alongside this guide to help parents with low motivation for change.
- Some parents may need referrals for additional individual or couples treatment.

CHAPTER 1

Module 1: Psychoeducation and Theoretical Foundations

(Recommended Length: 1 or 2 Sessions)

Materials Needed for the Module

Forms, parent summaries, worksheets, and handouts appear in Appendix A: Client Materials, located at the end of this therapist guide. You may photocopy this material for your clients, or you may download these items from the Programs That Work Web site at www.oxfordclinicalpsych. com/ADHDparenting. For a therapist outline of this and all modules, go to Appendix B: Therapist Outlines.

Parent Materials

- Module 1 Parent Summary
- Worksheet 1.1: ADHD in Families
- Worksheet 1.2: Looking at Connections: My Mood/Stress and How I Feel as a Caregiver
- Form A: Top Problems, to be given during the first session
- Form B: Top Problems, to be given at the start of each session beginning with Session 2

Therapist Note

Handouts can be distracting to parents when they are given during the session. The parent may read the handout rather than listen to the therapist. For this reason, you may wish to refrain from giving most handouts to the parent until the very end of the session, unless the handout or worksheet has a graphic or information that would be helpful to review or complete together in session.

Overall Module 1 Goals and Rationale

During Module 1, parents are oriented to the program and learn about the foundations of the intervention. This is a time to build rapport, learn more about the specific problems the child is having, identify treatment goals, and instill hope. Parents learn about several different models in Module 1, including (1) the ABC model of child behavior and (2) the transactional model of attention-deficit/hyperactivity disorder (ADHD) and families. The difficulties that children with ADHD experience are hard for parents to manage and can lead to parent stress and/or more frequent negative reactions to their child. It's easy to see how these child characteristics can lead parents to feel frustrated, stressed, worried, and/or sad about their child's behavior. This can make parents blame themselves or feel they're not doing a good job. On the other hand, some of our research shows that the degree to which a parent is responsive and sensitive can help or hinder temperamentally at-risk infants and young children in terms of the later development of ADHD symptoms (Miller, Degnan, et al., 2019). Teaching parents more effective ways to respond to their difficult child can have very important implications for the child's ongoing development. The ABC model of child behavior shared in Module 1 helps parents to begin to understand common cycles or traps that can happen when responding to their child's behavior and how to shift out of these cycles.

Parents also are introduced to mood monitoring and home practice assignments in Module 1. The importance of home practice assignments and the expectation for completing weekly home practice will be emphasized to make sure that parents know what to expect from treatment and how change will occur. Families often have beliefs about their child's behavior that lead them to underestimate their ability to influence their child's functioning. Understanding and addressing these beliefs early in the program can help with engagement and positive expectations of treatment.

> **Therapist Note**
>
> As discussed in the introduction to this therapist guide, this program assumes that the child is not present at sessions. However, there may be some cases in which you may wish to have the child present to practice certain skills, and this program allows for such flexibility.

Specific goals for this module include

- **Goal 1:** Orient and welcome parents to the program.
- **Goal 2:** Identify Top Problems and introduce parents to completing this assessment at the beginning of every session.
- **Goal 3:** Discuss the transactional model of ADHD and families, and encourage parents to identify factors that apply to their family.
- **Goal 4:** Introduce the ABC model of child behavior.
- **Goal 5:** Introduce monitoring mood and tracking parent feelings as a caregiver.

Module 1 Content (Divided by Goals)

Goal 1: Orient and welcome parents to the program

Welcome parents to the program and do introductions. You will start by providing them with some expectations for how the program will proceed. The program will focus on helping parents be and feel effective in their role as a parent of a child with ADHD as well as help parents manage their own stress and take care of themselves given the demands of parenting. By reducing stress and enhancing parents' self-regulation, it will help them to be more proactive and less reactive in their parenting. You will help parents understand why both of these areas (parenting and managing their own stress) are important and influence each other.

You can say something like,

> *In our meetings we will focus on two important things: (1) **helping you to be and feel effective in your role as a parent**; and (2) **helping you manage your stress and take care of yourself**. When you feel effective as a parent, your mood/stress level improves. When your mood/*

stress management and self-care improve, you are able to be a more effective parent. Both of these areas are important and influence each other!

> **Group Option:** Go over group rules, including confidentiality, avoiding negative talk, ensuring an equal opportunity to speak, and staying on task. Group members should also introduce themselves, provide brief information about their child, and then answer an icebreaker question, such as asking about something they like about their child or something they like to do with their child. Pointing out shared experiences among group members can enhance connection among group members and normalize their thoughts, feelings, and behaviors related to parenting a child with ADHD. It is important to keep these introductions brief as talkative parents can stretch this out! Group members will have plenty of time to get to know one another more over the course of the program.

The introduction to the program is a good time to validate the parents' experience of stress and the challenges of parenting a child with ADHD. It can be helpful to say that it would be hard to find a parent who is not experiencing significant stress with the demands of parenting a child with ADHD!

> *Goal 2: Identify "Top Problems" and introduce parents to completing this assessment at the beginning of every session*

The aim of this assessment is to have a client-driven measure of what their most important problems are and a method of tracking progress on addressing those problems during treatment (Weisz et al., 2011). Ask the parent what their three Top Problems are regarding their child. Write these down on Form A: Top Problems (located in Appendix A at the end of this therapist guide), in the parent's words, but make sure they are concrete, behavioral descriptions. For example, if a parent says "Inattention," ask "What does that look like?" and "How would you know if it is getting better?" By asking those questions, you might arrive at, "He gets up every 5 minutes when he is doing homework, and assignments that should take 30 minutes end up taking an hour and a half." Then ask for the severity rating for each of the three problems. The following is a list of examples of some problems:

- Gets frustrated easily with schoolwork and directions and shuts down (stops working)
- Anger when she doesn't get what she wants or is told no (kicks doors, throws things, has a tantrum and falls on floor)
- Needs repeated directions and reminders to get going and stay on track with school work and daily routines
- Cannot sit still—gets up from the dinner table and runs around a lot
- She forgets what she needs to do, and I have to tell her the same thing over and over again
- He is always talking and interrupting me when I talk
- He shuts down when a task is too difficult and will not continue on the task

It is important to confirm that the problems are related to ADHD and/ or co-occurring behavior problems because that is what this program is designed to best address. If the Top Problems are unrelated to ADHD/ behavior problems, it may indicate that the parent has other treatment priorities and may not be a good fit for this program.

Some parents' Top Problems may involve their own behavior, thoughts, or feelings. The following is a list of examples of some problems that may be identified by the parent as a major focus of treatment:

- I lose my temper and become extremely emotional when my child misbehaves
- When my child gets in trouble at school, it makes me feel depressed or anxious
- I don't know how to support my child in being successful at school
- I don't have the energy to deal with my child's behavior

After the first session, you can give Form B: Top Problems (located in Appendix A) to the parent at the beginning of the session (or when they arrive in the waiting area) to quickly complete each week. You should pre-fill (write in) the Top Problems from Form A: Top Problems each time. Check in with the parent about any major changes in the severity of the problems reported, but this does not need to be discussed every session or at length. As the parent progresses through the program, the

Top Problems may change and reassessment may be needed to ensure a shared sense of treatment goals.

Parents can write the three Top Problems chosen in this first session at the bottom of the Module 1 Parent Summary, located in Appendix A, at the end of this therapist guide.

> *Goal 3: Discuss the transactional model of ADHD and families, and encourage parents to identify factors that apply to their family*

Next, provide an overview of the transactional model of ADHD and families (there is more detailed information and background for the model in the Introduction). This model will help parents to gain a greater understanding of how parent characteristics and characteristics of the child interact to impact their relationship and the child's functioning across development. You will briefly review the six factors included in the model—Child Characteristics, Parent Characteristics, the Marital or Co-Parenting Relationship, the Sibling Relationship, School or Community Factors, and Culture—and the transactional relationships among them. You may find that having a whiteboard is helpful during this part of the session to write down factor headings and a few examples as you discuss. At this point, hand out Worksheet 1.1: ADHD in Families, located in Appendix A at the end of this therapist guide. Parents can begin to fill out this worksheet during the discussion (as an in-session activity) and complete it at home.

To introduce the model and first factor, you can say something like,

> *Now we are going to talk about a number of factors that interact to influence your child's and your family's functioning over time. The first factor is **Child Characteristics**. Your child's temperament (or personality) influences the way your child approaches and reacts to the world. Some children are born with more difficult temperaments, whereas other children are more easygoing. Temperament is seen from a very early age and can be thought of as the building blocks to the child's personality that are relatively stable tendencies over the long term.*

This is important to emphasize as research shows that temperament interacts with parenting to later predict ADHD symptoms (Miller, Degnan, et al., 2019). Thus, although temperament is considered relatively stable, experiences (such as parenting quality) can impact the stability of temperament and ultimately the child's long-term adjustment.

In this way, temperament does not impose a "life sentence"; rather, it is malleable. For example, parents can, indeed, help a fussy child learn to regulate. This will be an important point to emphasize.

The discussion with the parent should focus on the child's underlying temperamental style. For example, as an infant, the child may have been fussy and harder to get on a schedule, rather than being easy to soothe/calm and predictable. When a child is more emotional or cannot regulate themselves as well, parents may see behaviors like yelling, crying, and aggression. Another example may be how easygoing the child is ("goes with the flow") versus having problems with transitions or changes in routine ("more sensitive"). The information about ADHD provided in the Introduction to this therapist guide can be incorporated as needed as you help the parents to describe their child's characteristics. An example of this would be relating the parents' description of the child being "more sensitive" to the biological basis of ADHD and how it impacts their child's functioning. When a child has a harder time with transitions or change, parents will see more behaviors like tantrums and getting "stuck" on wanting things to be a certain way. If parents have more than one child, they can likely identify differences in the temperaments of their children.

Ask the parent to describe their child's temperament/personality and how that is related to child behaviors. You can also ask questions about other child factors that can influence child behavior.

- *Did your child have delays in talking, walking, or other developmental milestones? Any toilet training problems?*
- *Does your child have any health or physical problems that influence their behavior?*
- *Any problems with sleeping or eating?*
- *Does your child have difficulty regulating (or managing) their emotions?*
- *Any difficulties with friendships or social skills in general?*

Therapist Note

Children with ADHD often have difficulties with sleep, and strategies to address this are discussed in Module 3.

If parents have not yet discussed their child's ADHD symptoms (e.g., problems with attention span, activity level, impulse control), make sure to incorporate these in the discussion.

To introduce **Parent Characteristics** as the second factor in the model, you can say something like,

We adults also bring something to the table in our interactions with our children. Like children, caregivers have certain traits, such as being slow or quick to anger, emotional or mental health problems, flexibility, energy level, and health problems. Parts of our own characteristics can make parenting a difficult child even harder. For example, if you are very organized and cautious, a child with hyperactivity may be harder to deal with but this characteristic will also help you stick to the routines your child needs to thrive. Or, you may be more spontaneous (meaning that you don't usually plan ahead) and have a hard time sticking to routines, which may make parenting less stressful but also make it harder for you to stick to routines that your child may need.

These examples help parents to see that their own characteristics are often not all "good" or "bad" and to recognize how their own characteristics influence their experience as a parent.

Ask the parent to share a few of their own characteristics that influence parent–child interactions. Other parent characteristics that may influence interactions with their child include

- Executive functioning (e.g., difficulty organizing, planning, remembering, being flexible)
- Health or physical problems (e.g., insomnia, migraines, chronic health condition, physical disability)
- Parental cognitions (e.g., cognitive styles such as pessimism or anxiety)
- Parent mental health (e.g., problems with depression, anxiety, adult ADHD, alcohol/substance use)
- Emotion regulation (e.g., easily stressed, upset, angered)

Therapist Note

You can use questions from the Interpersonal Mindfulness in Parenting Scale (IMPS; Duncan, 2007) here to facilitate discussion, such as, "When I'm upset with my child, I notice how I am feeling before I take action" or "I rush through activities with my child without being really attentive to him/her."

Now you can go through the rest of the factors in a similar way. The third factor is the **Marital or Co-Parenting Relationship**. Conflict between parents can influence child functioning, and, likewise, child behavior problems can influence co-parenting and marital satisfaction. Parent stress can increase when interactions about the child with the co-parent or other family members are negative. One parent may experience the child's negative behavior more often than another. Parents often have different styles and may not agree on how to handle misbehavior, which can impact how they get along and communicate.

If there is a co-parent, ask if there is anything that would be helpful for you to know regarding this relationship and how it may influence the parent's experience of stress and parenting their child with ADHD.

The fourth factor is the **Sibling Relationship**. Children with ADHD typically have increased levels of conflict with their siblings, especially if the child with ADHD has co-occurring behavior problems (such as oppositional defiant or conduct disorder). Siblings of children with ADHD are also at an increased likelihood to have ADHD symptoms themselves. Siblings may also become resentful if they feel like their sister or brother with ADHD gets more parental attention. However, a strong, positive sibling relationship may act as a buffer against negative outcomes that children with ADHD often experience.

If there is a sibling (or other children living in the house), you can acknowledge that in families with multiple children there are many different relationships in one house. Ask parents how sibling relationships are going right now. You can explain that the skills parents will learn in the program can be used with siblings and to improve sibling interactions. Parents may express that they do not have as much time with other children, given the demands of parenting their child with ADHD. You can take note of this and help parents achieve goals with siblings as well as you go through future modules (e.g., scheduling a pleasant activity with a sibling or doing Special Time with a sibling).

The fifth factor is **School or Community Factors**. Schools and communities differ in terms of the level of support or stress they provide. Stressors can take many forms. Some families with whom you work may be struggling due to socioeconomic disadvantage and/or neighborhood violence. Other children live in communities or go to schools where there is increased stress due to high expectations for success across academics and extracurricular activities (which can be extra stressful for a child with ADHD who struggles academically and/or socially).

Ask parents how things are going for their child at school and how well they feel they can communicate with their child's school. Parents may have a lot to share about stress related to their experience with their child's school and the child's academic functioning. Because you have a lot to cover in this module, you can let them know that future sessions will be dedicated to helping their child with behavior at school and helping the parent to effectively communicate with the school.

The sixth factor is **Culture**. Parenting and expectations for child behavior occur within the cultural context. Views and stigma regarding mental health also vary according to culture. We have found that it is helpful to have an open conversation with the parent about these issues in this first session and throughout treatment. For example, grandparents and extended family may have opinions about the child's behavior and/or how to parent that can contribute added stress for the parent, and this may influence their reactions to the material included in this program.

By asking about cultural factors now and throughout the program, you can better understand beliefs and factors that may influence the acceptability or use of the strategies for parenting a child with ADHD and stress management. This is especially important when extended family is routinely involved in the child's care.

Interactions Among These Factors

All of the factors just described interact with one another to influence the child's adjustment over time (refer back to Figure I.1). Together, these interactive factors contribute to how impaired the child is with regard to their ADHD, as well as the extent to which the child adapts successfully or has increased difficulties (e.g., comorbid depression or conduct problems) over time.

To end this discussion, you can say something like,

> *Throughout this program, we will consider these factors for your family and how they interact to help you make changes in the Top Problems you identified today as well as related challenges that impact your child's and family's functioning.*

Stressors

You can also check in with the parents about any stressors that may be influencing their own current functioning, such as work or financial problems; relationship issues with other family members, friends, or their other children; transportation; child care; and so on.

> *Our mood and stress level at any given time also impact our parenting, and our child's behavior can impact our mood/stress in a transactional way. When your mood is down or you are feeling stressed out, it is (1) harder to be positive with your child; (2) easier to be negative, critical, or cranky with your child and other family members (e.g., the partner/co-parent); and (3) easier to give up or give in to your child rather than following through. This may create a cycle in which you see more misbehavior from your child, and then your mood becomes more down, your stress increases, and family relationships suffer.*

You can draw the diagram illustrated in Figure 1.1 on a whiteboard to illustrate this concept.

Goal 4: Introduce the ABC model of child behavior

As discussed in the introduction, the ABC model of child behavior is one of the foundations of this program. You will refer back to this model throughout the program as parents learn different strategies that target each of the ABC components. It is helpful during this initial discussion to write A-B-C on the board in a column and then write what each letter stands for and key points.

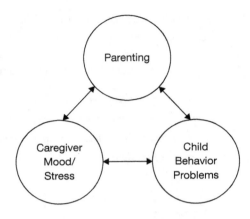

Figure 1.1

Simplified transactional model of parent–child interactions.

Today we are also going to talk about the ABCs of Child Behavior. The ABCs help us to understand the parts of a situation that affect your child's behavior.

A = Antecedents: The situations, settings, or people that impact the likelihood of your child behaving in a certain way. Your child's behavior can change depending on the situation.

- *Antecedents include things like home versus school, different classrooms, whether the child is in small versus large groups, which parent the child is with, one-on-one with an adult or not, etc.*
- *Antecedents can also include things such as the child's current mood, energy level, or irritability; parents' own current mood or energy level; the expectations or rules that are given when entering a situation; and other characteristics of the setting or people involved.*
- *Elicit examples from the parent about situations where their child does their best and situations where the child has the most challenges.*
- *Thinking about antecedents helps you to set your child up for success.*

B = Child Behavior: The observable ways your child acts; what they do.

- *Behaviors can be positive or negative. In this program, you will help parents identify behaviors that they want their child to change or improve.*

- *It is very important to be specific about the behaviors parents want their child to change. For example, parents may say that they want their child to "behave better/be good," but that is very general. What does "be good" mean? You can help parents to define more specific behaviors that can be easily observed, like "following a direction the first time the child is asked," "giving another child a turn with a toy or game," or "sitting down to start homework at the designated time."*

C = Consequences: Consequences happen after the behavior and influence whether the behavior will happen again.

- *Parents often think the word "consequence" means punishment. Explain that consequences are any responses that follow behavior, both positive and negative. Positive consequences increase the chances parents will see a behavior again. Negative consequences decrease the chances parents will see a behavior again.*
- *Examples of positive consequences include parent attention or access to a privilege, like playing on a tablet or watching television. Parents will want to give positive consequences after behaviors that they want to increase, like completing homework or following directions.*
- *A challenging aspect of explaining consequences is that sometimes parents intend for a consequence to be negative (like telling their child what they are doing is wrong), but the consequence is actually positive for the child (because the child is getting adult attention which "fuels" the behavior).*

Adult attention is very rewarding for kids! Attention is like potato chips—you may prefer one type over another, but in general you won't turn down potato chips! Although your child prefers positive attention, your negative attention is often better than no attention at all. Another helpful analogy is that "child behavior is like your car—you don't pay much attention to your car unless it isn't working." Child behavior you want to decrease (like arguing) is likely to keep happening if you attend to it—even if the attention you are giving is negative or corrective. We want to make sure our attention is given most when a child is behaving in ways that we want to see more of because of the power of our attention. We'll talk a lot more about this throughout the program.

Ask parents to give a few examples of what positive or negative consequences they are using currently. During the discussion you can review the following concepts and ask the questions provided to help parents understand the connection between consequences and the likelihood that a behavior will happen again:

- Children may misbehave to gain a positive consequence, like parent attention, or keep misbehaving until parents "give in" (e.g., allowing them to stay up later or to get a desired treat). You can ask, "*What are some ways that your child may inadvertently be rewarded (get something desirable) when they misbehave?*"

- Children may also misbehave to escape from something that is unpleasant, boring, or effortful, like throwing a tantrum to get out of homework, cleaning up, or going to bed (so there is a "positive" consequence, getting out of something or extending bedtime). You can ask the parent about some things that their child gets to escape or avoid when they misbehave. If the parent has a difficult time coming up with examples, you can discuss homework or chores as an example.

- Often, parents will say that they feel like positive and negative consequences don't seem to affect their child's behavior and that nothing they have tried works for them. Children do not need to be successful in avoiding unpleasant activities or gaining positive consequences all of the time to maintain disruptive or noncompliant behavior. It is similar to an adult's gambling habit. A person will continue gambling even though they only get payoffs every once in a while. Even if a child only gets out of doing their chores once a week, they will act up every day with the hope of getting out of doing chores. One way to explain the power of inconsistent reinforcement is to say, "*If your child's misbehavior works once in a while to get out of something, you will keep seeing that misbehavior. This is the same principle that explains why people keep putting money in a slot machine even though they don't win much of the time. If there is any chance it will work, they will keep trying. Consistency is key in changing your child's behavior so that they learn and change their behavior in the long run!*" You can share with parents that many things impact our consistency, including the intensity of the child's reactions and the parent's own characteristics and stressors. That is why this program helps families address many aspects of family functioning to help set them up for success.

Therapist Note

Throughout this therapist guide, we will include an ABC icon to remind you to tie the material back to the ABC model when appropriate.

After this discussion, give the parent the Module 1 Parent Summary (see Appendix A) and explain that they will receive a summary for each module to help them remember key concepts. You can show them that there is a place to write the three Top Problems chosen today.

Goal 5: Introduce monitoring mood and tracking parent feelings as a caregiver

Mood monitoring allows for the identification of patterns in how mood varies over time. By monitoring their mood, parents can begin to see connections between their mood and other aspects of their life (including their parenting). Throughout this program, parents will be asked to monitor their mood and then other aspects of their life (activities, thoughts, and so on). The mood monitoring in this module serves as the foundation for all of those activities.

> *Because we are going to be talking about your mood/stress and caregiving, for this week I'd like you to start paying more attention to your mood/stress and how you feel about your parenting. Sometimes it helps to monitor or keep track of your mood on a regular basis to see what is happening that contributes to positive or negative mood.*

You can then hand out Worksheet 1.2: Looking at Connections: My Mood/Stress and How I Feel as a Caregiver and explain:

- *Each day, parents will rate their mood on a 1–10 scale (1 being the worst they have ever felt, 5 neither good nor bad, 10 the best they've ever felt). You can ask the parent to give their mood rating right in this moment to show how quick/easy it can be.*
- *Parents will also rate how they felt about their caregiving each day on a 1–10 scale (1 being the worst day they ever had as a caregiver, 5 an okay day, 10 the ideal parenting day). Ask the parent to give their rating right in this moment of how they feel as a caregiver.*
- *It is important that parents try to complete the ratings around the same time each day (e.g., before bed).*

- *Some people prefer to do their mood monitoring on their mobile phones rather than filling out paper forms, which is perfectly fine. There are now many free mobile applications available for mood monitoring. Parents should use whichever system they feel most comfortable with and that they can be most consistent with.*

Home Practice

At the end of the first session, introduce home practice (or homework) to the parent.

Most weeks, you will be asked to practice *something outside of our sessions. It's the regular practice that makes change happen. Talking about the concepts and strategies here is just the very start. Applying the concepts and strategies to your life on a consistent basis is* essential *for long-term change in your mood/stress, parenting, and child's behavior.*

Home practice for this module is:

- Monitoring mood and how the parent feels as a caregiver (Worksheet 1.2: Looking at Connections: My Mood/Stress and How I Feel as a Caregiver).

Group Option: Ask for a few volunteers to state when they think they will do the daily mood ratings and how they will remember to do it. Building the home practice into their routine (e.g., after putting their children to bed) can be helpful.

CHAPTER 2

Module 2: Special Time and Pleasant Activities Scheduling

(Recommended Length: 1 or 2 Sessions)

Materials Needed for the Module

Forms, parent summaries, worksheets, and handouts appear in Appendix A: Client Materials, located at the end of this therapist guide. You may photocopy this material for your clients, or you may download these items from the Treatments ThatWork web site at www.oxfordclinicalpsych.com/ ADHDparenting. For an outline of this and all modules, go to Appendix B: Therapist Outlines.

Parent Materials

- Module 2 Parent Summary
- Worksheet 2.1: Special Time Record Form
- Worksheet 2.2: Pleasant Activities
- Worksheet 2.3: Looking at Connections: My Mood/Stress, Caregiving, and Activities
- Handout 2.1: Special Time Guidelines

Assessment to Be Given at Every Session

- Form B: Top Problems

Given the importance of home practice, it is critical to take a few minutes to review parents' practice since the last session. Taking time for this review each week not only conveys the importance of home practice but also helps to troubleshoot any problems they encountered with prior skills before covering new material. Note that this can be done in either an individual or group format.

In Module 1, parents learned how parent and child functioning are connected through the ABC model and the transactional model of ADHD and families for child behavior. Parents were also introduced to regularly monitoring their mood and their feelings about their parenting. The following questions can be used during the home practice review:

- *Did you think more about the child, parent, and/or other environmental factors that can make interactions more difficult in your family?*
- *How about stressors that affect you and your child?*
- *How did the mood monitoring go? Did you remember to do it? What helped you remember? Did you notice any patterns in your mood?*
- *Did you notice a connection between your mood and your parenting? How about your mood and your child's behavior?*
- *If you didn't do the mood monitoring consistently, what got in the way? How can you remember to do this over the next week?*

 Some parents will have a difficult time remembering to monitor their mood. Remind them to do their mood monitoring at the same time every day. They can use the strategy of "habit stacking" to tie the new habit of mood monitoring to something they already do at the end of the night (such as putting on their pajamas). You can encourage them to use their calendar or planner (electronic or paper form) to record their mood if this is easier than using your monitoring sheets. If they are using a calendar system on their mobile phone, they can also set a calendar reminder/alarm to remind them to complete mood monitoring. More information about calendar systems is provided in Module 3.

Therapist Note

Throughout this therapist guide, we will include a Calendar icon to indicate when parents may find it helpful to add an activity to their calendar.

Therapist Notes

Reminder: The importance of practice at home should be emphasized in each session. Families need continued reminders that the session time is spent covering information that will then be applied at home. You can use analogies that make sense to the family, such as going to the doctor for an antibiotic but then going and remembering to take it daily!

Note: Make sure to adjust the home practice review based on what was assigned in the previous session. If topics haven't been covered yet, omit the questions about that content from the home practice review. Also, if this home practice review does not include content that has been covered and assigned for home practice (e.g., if you are doing modules in a different order), make sure to expand the home practice review to include all assigned items.

Overall Module 2 Goals and Rationale

During Module 2, parents increase pleasant activities with their child and on their own. Parents of children with attention-deficit/hyperactivity disorder (ADHD) can easily get caught in the cycle of giving more corrective or negative feedback than positive feedback. This negative feedback loop can impact the parent–child relationship, the child's behavior, and the parent's mood. It can also impact interactions with co-parents and siblings, which further perpetuates negative cycles within the family. By the time they seek treatment, parents frequently say that they are finding it hard to enjoy time with their child with ADHD. Although they love their child, they sometimes find it hard to "like" them. In this module, you can instill hope that the parent can begin to enjoy time with their child again and ultimately improve their relationship.

Parents will learn strategies to positively attend to their child during a regular "Special Time." Special Time can then be used as an example of a pleasant activity in the cognitive-behavioral therapy (CBT) model that will positively influence parents' thoughts and feelings. Parents will also learn to identify and schedule pleasant activities they can do *without* their child to gain some respite from parenting and therefore improve their mood and enjoyment of time *with* their child(ren).

Many parents need to be "given permission" to participate in self-care activities away from their child and other work/family demands. In this program, parent self-care is an essential treatment component that is repeatedly emphasized. Pleasant activities are not viewed as optional, but rather as a necessary part of self-care that is an important component of meeting the demands of parenting a challenging child. Over the course of the program, one overarching goal is to help parents *prioritize* their self-care, for the sake of their own mental health and their family's well-being.

Therapist Note

Throughout this therapist guide, we will include a Self-Care icon to remind you to emphasize to the parent the importance of self-care.

Specific goals for this module include

- **Goal 1:** Teach parents about the influence of their positive attention on the parent–child relationship and child behavior.
- **Goal 2:** Teach specialized attending strategies for parents to have a consistent daily Special Time with their child.
- **Goal 3:** Introduce the CBT model and the idea of increasing parents' engagement in pleasant activities to improve their own mood so that they can ultimately be in a better place to parent their child with ADHD.
- **Goal 4:** Identify the most mood-enhancing pleasant activities that the parent can add to their schedule in the short and long term.
- **Goal 5:** Introduce the idea of tracking pleasant activities and mood to better understand the connection between the two.

Goal 1: Teach parents about the influence of their positive attention on the parent–child relationship and child behavior

Children with ADHD need a special "dose" of consistent positive attention that other children may not need to the same degree to stay motivated and behave appropriately (think orchid vs. dandelion!). At the same time, it can be easy for parents of children with ADHD to fall into the trap of correcting their child's behavior and providing a high degree of negative feedback—such challenging child behavior "pulls for" these parenting responses. However, the child's behavior problems make it both *more challenging and more necessary* to give a consistent "higher dosage" of positive attention. Indeed, years of research have shown that positive parenting (e.g., praise and a warm parent–child relationship) can protect against negative long-term outcomes for children with ADHD, such as depression, conduct problems, and substance use (e.g., Chronis et al., 2007). For many families, it can be challenging to have a good time together and maintain a warm, positive relationship when the child has frequent difficult behaviors. As the therapist, you should normalize this reaction because many parents express guilt for feeling this way. You will explain to parents the benefits of having a daily Special Time with their child to help them enjoy time together (with few parental demands) on a regular basis, to improve their relationship, and to have their child view them as someone the child wants to spend time with and to "work for." This relationship will also be critical as the child moves into adolescence, when it will be essential for the teen to feel close enough to their parents to share problems and feelings that arise.

You may say something like this:

For many families, a child's ADHD and challenging behaviors can make it hard to have a good time together and maintain a positive relationship. We are going to talk about something you can do to improve your relationship with your child. It can be very hard to enjoy time with your child when they need a lot of correction, push limits, and are not able to do the things you expect them to do. Today you will learn how to do a daily "Special Time" activity with your child to help you have a good time together, improve your relationship, and help you influence your child's behavior in a positive way. This can help your relationship in the short term, and this is also important for the long term because you want your child to feel comfortable coming to you to share their thoughts, feelings, and problems in the tween and teenage years.

To help parents consider the impact of positive attention on someone's motivation to work and possibly the quality of work, ask them to think of the best and worst supervisors, mentors, coaches, or teachers they have had throughout their lives.[1] Have them consider how they felt about their supervisors and how much they wanted to work for them. Write down examples of the best and worst supervisor traits. You can add examples of traits if that is helpful. Examples of positive supervisor traits include being kind, helpful, considerate, fair, understanding, predictable, transparent, and encouraging. Examples of negative supervisor traits include being harsh, critical, demanding, inconsistent, dismissive, and absent.

You may say something like this:

Think about the best supervisor, mentor, coach, or teacher you've had. Now think about the worst. What words would you use to describe the best and worst supervisors you have had? How did you feel about these supervisors, and how did that influence your desire to work for them and consider their feedback? What qualities in a supervisor motivated you to work hard to get their approval?

Ask parents to consider if they feel that their child has gone "on strike" and is not working optimally. Their child's ADHD and co-occurring symptoms will impact their work; however, a parent's relationship with their child and the quality of their feedback will also influence their child's "work." Before the parent begins to implement strategies for changing their child's behavior, they will need to come to enjoy their time together again. They need to have more positive interactions to tip the scale away from negative interaction patterns that have developed. This provides the foundation for the rest of the work that will be done in this program.

---

[1] This is a common analogy used in several cognitive-behavioral treatments, including Barkley's parent training program (2013).

Children with ADHD and challenging behaviors often get more correc-
tive feedback and criticism from parents, teachers, and peers than praise
and encouragement. This can have long-term negative effects on the
child's mood and the way they think about themselves (their self-esteem).
It is stressful to parent a child with ADHD, and the scale can easily tip
toward more negative feedback, even though you don't intend for that to
happen. How do you think your child would describe you as a "super-
visor"? How might that influence how your child responds to you?

> *Goal 2: Teach specialized attending strategies for parents to have a*
> *consistent daily Special Time with their child*

How to Communicate During Special Time

The main goal of Special Time[2] is for the parent to *follow the child's
lead* during an activity the child chooses/enjoys. Parents will join their
child for an activity for about 10 minutes each day. Special Time may
initially seem simple, but it is indeed a very different way of interacting
that does not feel natural or comfortable for some parents. This can be a
function of a parent's culture or the way they themselves were parented,
or both. Other parents may feel like they are too busy for Special Time
and become impatient or distracted by other work/family demands.
Nevertheless, your goal is to help parents see the importance of Special
Time and do their best to follow the guidelines. In doing so, it may be
important to briefly discuss the parent's experience of being parented
and how things like parental praise are viewed in their culture/family.

> *During Special Time you will not take over the activity in any way, try to*
> *teach or instruct your child, or tell your child to do something. Your main*
> *job is simply to give your child your full attention (without distractions)*
> *and follow your child's lead. How does this fit with how you yourself were*
> *parented?*

During Special Time, parents will use ways of communicating with their
child that allow the child to be in the lead. Parents of younger children

---

[2] Special Time is used in behavioral parent training programs following the Hanf
model (Reitman & McMahon, 2013), including Barkley (2013), Eyberg and
Funderburk (2011), and others.

will *describe* what their child is doing (e.g., "You are stacking the blocks") to show interest and approval. Descriptions allow the parent to stay "a step behind" because the parent can't describe an action until the child has done it. In this way, the parent is truly following rather than guiding or directing where the play goes next.

Parents will also allow their child to stay in the lead by *avoiding questions*. Questions can indeed be used to show interest and can be a good teaching tool at other times, so some parents will not initially understand why we are asking them to avoid questions during Special Time. Parents often think their questions are nondirective, but questions can lead the conversation or lead the play in unintended ways. By avoiding questions, parents learn to wait for the child to say what they would like to share without any direction, pressure, or demands.

Let parents know that the frequency of talking during Special Time can depend on their child's age and interests. In general, younger children like more frequent and enthusiastic feedback, and older children prefer for their parent(s) to be more laid back and low-key during Special Time. For older children, constant talking can feel intrusive, and they can often sense praise that is not genuine or seems trite (e.g., "Great job drawing that circle" won't work as well with older children!). Taking a more relaxed pace can make the interactions appear more natural and reciprocal for older children.

During Special Time, you will watch and describe the things that your child does like a sports announcer. For younger children, you can do this more frequently and enthusiastically. For older children, you want to be a little more low-key. Describing your child's play is simply letting your child know that you are fully paying attention and interested in what they are doing, that you are 100% there with them. It is really important to give your child your full attention during Special Time.

Describing what your child is doing is not the same as asking your child questions. Asking questions can be a nice way of interacting with your child during other times; however, you want to avoid questions during Special Time. You want your child to lead the direction of conversation and play. Questions can lead your child in a different direction than they might go on their own.

Additionally, parents should *stay away from giving directions* during Special Time. Telling children what to do takes away their lead and can make the time together less enjoyable. It can be challenging to avoid this when children need information or when parents want to provide a correction. Parents can interact without giving directions by modeling how to do something (e.g., "I am writing the letter 'A,'" "I am drawing a straight line") to keep their child in the lead. You can reassure parents that providing instruction and giving children directions are important aspects of parenting, but they can do those things outside of Special Time.

Criticism should be avoided during Special Time as well. Critical statements take away from the positive nature of Special Time and can result in negative child behaviors. Often this comes up for parents in the form of pointing out mistakes that children make. Parents should be encouraged to only provide information instead of pointing out the mistake (e.g., saying "That is a teal bead," instead of "That is not a green bead on the bracelet, that is a teal bead.")

During Special Time, parents should *praise their child's positive behaviors.* This will be discussed in more detail in Module 4, but, at this point, encourage parents to praise those positive behaviors they notice during Special Time (e.g., "I like how you are playing so calmly with me," "You are working so carefully on your drawing"). Parents should try to be as specific as possible with their praise. You can tie in the supervisor analogy discussed earlier and the impact of positive feedback on how their child feels.

Ask parents to briefly list what they will do and not do during Special Time. Help them as needed to state that they will describe and praise, and they will not ask questions, direct, or criticize. Emphasize the overall goal of following their child's lead to help them have plenty of opportunities to give their child positive attention for a short time each day.

Scheduling Special Time and Appropriate Activities

Help parents to understand the importance of learning to relax (more on this in Module 5) during Special Time so they can provide genuine positive attention to their child without being distracted or less present by thinking of all the other things they have to do. It is best for parents to select a time when distractions are limited and to not have a television, laptop, or mobile phone nearby. If possible, they should also arrange to have Special Time when their other child(ren) are sleeping, otherwise occupied, or able to be watched by another caregiver. Encourage parents to join their child for activities that allow for them to not have to direct or control their child's behavior. That is, parents should avoid games with rules, homework, etc., that may pull for them to be directive.

You want to choose a time of day that is best for both you and your child, perhaps when other children are occupied with someone else or sleeping. Or at a time when your partner, spouse, or other caregiver can help with your other child(ren).

You should try to avoid watching television or playing with electronics together for Special Time because talking to your child during a show could be annoying to them and may model interrupting someone's activity. You also want to find things to describe about what your child is doing rather than just watching characters in a show. Building toys, art activities (that aren't too messy), and some sports activities (like soccer or basketball) are great for Special Time—any activity that allows your child to be creative and that you are able to let them lead without needing to give them directions or corrections.

Parents may want to set out several appropriate activities in advance of Special Time and then allow their child to choose from the activities. Keep in mind that activities appropriate for a younger child (e.g., playing with blocks, drawing with crayons) may not be as engaging for an older child. Crafts (e.g., pipe cleaners, modeling clay, spin art, making jewelry) and certain art supplies (e.g., gel pens, glitter glue, hole punches) can be successful in engaging older children. Other Special Time activities with older children could include making model cars, sand art, bracelets, or other creative activities. Construction toys such as Lego and K'Nex are often still appropriate for older children. Outside play, such as kicking the soccer ball, playing catch, or jumping on the trampoline, can also be good Special Time activities for older children. Cooperative board games can be a good option for some children.

Parents of older children will often ask about video games. If older children will not engage in other Special Time activities (therapists should always encourage parents to try out several other activities before choosing video games), parents can use video games as their Special Time activity as long as the video game is not violent and the parent is not competing against their child in the game. Games where parents can talk to their child and interact with them are best (e.g., Wii Sports, Minecraft Creative Mode).

Remember, the primary goal is to spend time with your child without criticizing, directing, or controlling your child's behavior. Instead, you are watching and appreciating what your child is doing.

Explore with parents *what message they are sending* to their children when they give their child their full attention and show genuine interest and appreciation. Help parents to make the connection that their child does not have to act out in order to be noticed.

How do you think your child will react to Special Time? Do you think it will help your child to learn that appropriate behavior is noticed and appreciated?

Also, help parents come to appreciate the potential *long-term impact* of spending Special Time with their child on a regular basis.

How do you think that prioritizing consistent Special Time in your schedule will affect your relationship with your child in the short and long term?

How to Handle Negative Behavior During Special Time

Children often demonstrate good behavior during Special Time because they have the lead, and the parent is not making demands and is showing lots of positive interest. Thus, as parents master the Special Time skills, their interactions during this time will usually be very pleasant. Ideally, this is also a one-on-one situation in which children with ADHD typically behave better. You can point this out as a good example of the "A" (or antecedent) in the ABC model of child behavior.

However, at the same time, we want the parent to be prepared for how to handle inappropriate behavior during Special Time if it occurs. To avoid giving negative attention, the parent should remove their attention until the unwanted behavior ends. You can use the ABC model (Module 1) to show that removing your attention for an attention-seeking behavior is a way to decrease that behavior (which will be explained in more detail in Module 3). However, parents should be prepared for the *extinction burst* that may occur when they first remove their attention (also discussed more in Module 3). If the child's behavior escalates to aggression or destruction during Special Time, then Special Time ends for the day. It is important for parents to understand that Special Time is *not* a privilege or reward. Special Time is never taken away for something that happens outside of Special Time. In fact, Special Time should be viewed like a vitamin or medication that can help the child (and parent) to get back on track. In essence, Special Time lays the foundation for positive and warm parent–child interactions that are necessary for the other skills to be most effective.

Your child is very likely to behave appropriately during Special Time given the one-on-one time that is positive and encouraging. However, if your child does something negative, like yell, play roughly, or say something inappropriate, briefly turn your attention away from your child and then turn back when the behavior has stopped. If the negative behavior continues/escalates to something like aggression or breaking something, tell your child that the Special Time has ended because of their behavior and they will have another chance for Special Time tomorrow. Your child will learn the difference between behaviors that get your positive attention and behaviors you turn away from. When you turn away to remove attention for minor unwanted behaviors, keep your face very neutral. We know this may be hard when your child is acting inappropriately. In future meetings will talk more about keeping-calm (CBT) skills that you can use in these situations.

Also, Special Time is a therapeutic support for your child (like medication or exercise), not a privilege. Thus, Special Time should never be taken away for behaviors that occur outside of Special Time. In fact, when a child is having a more challenging day with behavior, Special Time is an opportunity to have a positive influence on your child's behavior.

Often children will not want Special Time to end. Parents should acknowledge that they, too, enjoy Special Time and don't want to see it end, but then reassure the child that they will have Special Time again tomorrow.

Role-Play the Special Time Strategies

Demonstrate in a role-play how to follow a child's lead in a play activity, using descriptions and praise and avoiding questions and criticism. Show how to turn away or remove attention for an inappropriate behavior and then to give attention back as soon as possible for a neutral or positive behavior.

Introduce Worksheet 2.1: Special Time Record Form

Show parents the Special Time Record Form they will use this week. Have them share when they think they can do Special Time and how they will remember to do it. Building the time into their typical routine (e.g., always doing Special Time after dinner or before bed—habit stacking!) can be helpful to make this a family routine (see Module 3). It is also helpful for the parent to add Special Time to their calendar system (calendars will also be elaborated on in Module 3). Help the parent to problem-solve any barriers, including when to do it and what activities may work best. See "Parent Reactions to Special Time" for ideas to handle a variety of parent reactions, either in this session or when they return and discuss how their initial attempts to do Special Time went.

You can use this form (show Worksheet 2.1: Special Time Record Form) to record your practice, how it goes this week, and how you feel during Special Time. When will you and your child be available to spend this time together? What activities does your child enjoy that you can join? Make sure to think of some activities that are feasible to do on a typical day in your household. You want to make it easy for you to do this on a regular basis.

Parent Reactions to Special Time

Parents can have a variety of reactions to the idea of beginning to have consistent Special Time with their child. Common reactions and ideas for addressing them include the following:

- Parents may remark that the play techniques seem especially simple and easy to implement. In fact, not directing the child or asking questions and fully concentrating on describing and praising are *very challenging skills* for some caregivers and take considerable practice for most parents to do well.
- Some parents may note that they are *too busy* for this sort of activity. Encourage them to *make time*, that this (facilitating a warm and positive parent–child relationship) is indeed a *priority* and that the techniques will take time to practice and master but will eventually lead to positive outcomes if used consistently. After all, having a positive relationship with their children is a priority or they would not be seeking help. Use motivational strategies when necessary to remind parents of how important doing something they haven't been doing is for the possibility of change (in the Introduction for further details on how to use motivational interviewing [MI]).
- Some children may also need time to get used to their parents communicating in a different way. Although these strategies are designed to have a positive impact, it is not uncommon for children (especially older children) to say things like "why are you talking like that?" or "stop saying that" when a parent begins to do Special Time. As the parent's attending skills become more natural and the child gets used to a bigger dose of their parent's positive attention, these reactions should disappear. The majority of children truly enjoy having their parent's full attention. It can take time for some children to learn that it is their appropriate (vs. inappropriate) behavior that will earn their parent's interest and approval. Some children may feel uncomfortable at first with a change in their parent's

behavior, even if it is a positive one. Ultimately, children will find their parent's positive attention far more reinforcing than their negative attention.

- Caregivers may feel silly or awkward doing this activity. Again, if they take time to master this, it will begin to feel normal and eventually contribute to seeing less negative child behavior.
- Caregivers may ask whether they should tell the child about Special Time. For younger children, it can help to tell them it is their Special Time and that it will happen each day (or most days). For older children, parents may wish not to "schedule" Special Time and simply join their child for play when there is a good opportunity to do so each day.
- Parents may express that their child with ADHD already receives "too much" of their time and attention and may have concerns about siblings getting even less of their time. Let them know that you understand these concerns and how these concerns may be a significant part of why the family presented for treatment. Express the belief that Special Time will have therapeutic benefits that will help the parent feel better about the time they are spending with their child with ADHD, and remind them that these strategies can be used with siblings as well.

Address any concerns in general that parents have about the appropriateness of play with their child or concerns about the reactions of other family members to this technique. Some parents will need help identifying activities that their child would like them to join. Parents may also predict that the child will prefer to interact with other kids in the family rather than one-on-one with the parent, or parents may be concerned about siblings feeling jealous. You can remind parents that they are practicing a different way of interacting with their child with ADHD, which will make the one-on-one time more desirable. It's also important to remember that although their child will be playing, this is actually a therapeutic time for the family.

You can also help parents to problem-solve issues with their other children, such as giving each child Special Time if possible, or doing Special Time when a sibling is napping/asleep, at school, or engaged in a desired activity so they are less likely to interrupt. If there is a co-parent in the household, they can trade off doing Special Time with the child(ren).

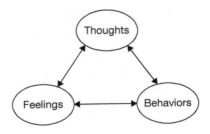

Figure 2.1

Cognitive-behavioral therapy model.

> *Goal 3: Introduce the CBT model and the idea of increasing parents' engagement in pleasant activities to improve their own mood so that they can ultimately be in a better place to parent their child with ADHD*

Special Time is an opportunity to add a *positive action* and to work on *tipping the balance* between positive and negative experiences in both the parent's and child's lives and their relationship. You will discuss how increasing pleasant activities (what you *do*) changes how you *think* and *feel* by introducing the CBT model (which we also refer to as the "thoughts-feelings-behaviors triangle" in this therapist guide), as illustrated in Figure 2.1.

Draw the CBT model on the board or on a piece of paper and give definitions for thoughts, feelings, and behaviors:

> *Feelings are our emotions, such as happiness, stress, sadness, frustration, and so on. Behavior is how we act, what we do, and say. When we feel good, we may say something nice or give a hug. When we are stressed or down, we may complain, yell, cry, nag, or talk less. Thoughts are what we say to ourselves; how we think about ourselves, other people, and situations. When we feel good we may assume the best, focus on the positive, or see a problem as solvable. When we are stressed or down, we have more thoughts that are negative or critical about ourselves, our parenting, our child, and others (e.g., our spouse). We tend to focus on wanting to feel better but it's really hard to just will ourselves to feel a different way. It is usually easiest to change behavior in order to change how we feel and think, so we will start with that. Later we will talk about changing what you say to yourself (your thinking) to change how we feel and act.*

Doing Special Time with your child is an example of a pleasant activity/ positive action that can have an impact on your mood (and your child's mood!). This action can influence both your thoughts and your feelings about your child and your parenting, which in turn can impact your child's mood, thoughts, and behaviors.

On the CBT model, draw an arrow pointing from behavior to feelings. Also draw an arrow from behavior to thoughts. Ask the parent what thoughts they may have about their child or self during Special Time. You can also draw an arrow from behavior to feelings and point out that this positive action may result in more relaxed feelings because, during Special Time, the parent does not need the child to do something or stop doing something or teach the child something. You can say something like,

Imagine that your child had a tough day at school and what thoughts and feelings you might have when you receive the feedback from the teacher. You then engage in Special Time that evening with your child (an action). How would this action influence your thoughts and feelings about your child? How would this action influence your thoughts and feelings about yourself as a parent? How might Special Time impact your child's thoughts, feelings, and behaviors after a rough day at school?

Next, expand the discussion to include the importance of pleasant activities that are *not* with their child and do not involve parenting demands. So often, parents put their own needs *after* their child(ren)'s or do not consider their own needs at all. This may be especially true for parents of children with emotional or behavioral health concerns; however, it is for these families that parent self-care is *even more* important. Parenting a child with ADHD can be viewed as a chronic stressor, and self-care is absolutely essential for parents' mental health! Help the parent to understand that focusing on their own self-care will give them the emotional resources to best meet the demands of providing the support their child needs.

As we talked about before, there are days when you don't feel very well— you might be stressed or down or nervous or cranky or overwhelmed. If you are down or stressed, it can be hard to parent the way that you want to.

Today we are going to talk about ways to take time on a regular basis to do the things that you enjoy or to fit some enjoyable activities into your already-busy daily routine.

Remember, often "behavior" is the easiest part of the thoughts-feelings-behavior model to change. By changing our behavior, we can change our feelings and thoughts.

It is easy to get into a cycle where you have so much to do ("have-to's") that you have little time for the "want-to's."

You might feel guilty for doing anything for yourself (because your family or kids need you), and while you certainly have a lot of demands on your time, we are going to suggest that taking time for you will benefit your family in the long run. It also benefits your family because if you are taking care of yourself, you have more to give to them. Therefore, in this program, I would like to make doing the activities you enjoy a priority for you. It may help to imagine what you would say to a friend or to your child about the importance of spending some time doing things they enjoy.

Some parents really do have too much on their plates and require some help with assertiveness or saying no. These skills are presented in Module 6, but relate here as they can be helpful in allowing parents to create more time to do the things they most enjoy.

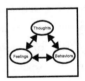

Therapist Note

Throughout this therapist guide, we will include a CBT model icon to remind you to tie the material back to this model when appropriate.

Goal 4: Identify the most mood-enhancing pleasant activities that the parent can add to their schedule in the short and long term

Using Worksheet 2.2: Pleasant Activities, you will help parents to generate a list of activities that they find enjoyable in the areas that are important to them (e.g., friends/family, health and wellness, career, spirituality; these life areas are drawn from Lejuez, Hopko, & Hopko, 2001). The goal is for parents to identify 3–5 pleasant activities that are feasible to do on a regular basis, important to them, and likely to be enjoyable.

We are now going to talk about pleasant activities that you can add to your schedule. For ideas, take a look at Worksheet 2.2: Pleasant Activities (give parent the form). You will want to increase activities that you find enjoyable in the areas that are important to you. You should select one or two activities in each area that you can aim to start or do more frequently. These activities should be very specific and simple like "calling my sister once per week" or "going to church on Sunday." These activities should be consistent with things you value most, so if your friendships are important to you, spending more time with friends is a good goal. If your health and fitness are important to you, choose activities related to this area of your life. These should be activities that are both important to you and that you enjoy. Your goals should also be very specific in order to increase the likelihood that you will actually do them.

Therapist Note

Different activities can influence mood for different people so encourage parents to stay open and experiment to see what is most helpful. Activities that fall in the areas of social, mastery (gaining/improving a skill, completing a task), contributing, and physical activities can be especially mood enhancing (Lewinsohn, Munoz, Youngren, & Zeiss, 1986).

There may also be activities that make you feel good that do not take too much additional time in your daily routine, such as listening to your favorite music, an audiobook, or podcasts on your daily commute without the kids; having your favorite meal for dinner; using a special shower gel; lighting a scented candle; treating yourself to a special tea or coffee; or calling a friend or family member. Many of these activities can be done while you are showering, working, driving, or doing household chores so they really do not have to "cost" you any time. Even though you may already be doing some of these things, simply changing the way you think about or savor these activities can make it feel like a more pleasant activity for you. In other words, be in the moment when you're doing these activities, rather than thinking about all of the other things you have to do. In addition, you may find that devoting time to something like reading or a hobby also leads to more positive social interactions because you can talk about these things that interest you with others.

When you decide on a specific activity that is (1) able to be added to your schedule, (2) important to you, and (3) something you think you would enjoy, write it down on Worksheet 2.2. If you are having a hard time thinking of activities, just remember that you don't always have to do things that you have done before or used to do. Sometimes spending time in a new activity can be just as rewarding. Choose things that you can do on a daily, weekly, and monthly basis to get the most benefits, and choose a good range of activities.

Things that help with planning include (1) scheduling the activity on your calendar (treat it like any other appointment and set an alarm to remind you to do it), (2) scheduling an activity with others (accountability helps), and (3) having a back-up plan in case something comes up and you have to do a different activity (e.g., if you plan to go on a walk with your neighbor but it is storming outside).

Group Option: As parents are completing Worksheet 2.2: Pleasant Activities, it can help to have them work together to generate ideas and solutions. Ask each person to share with the group one or two activities they are going to do in the coming weeks, how it might fit into their schedule, and how they will remember to do it.

Therapist Note

Parents may seem overwhelmed and express that there are simply too many barriers and not enough time in their day to schedule pleasant activities for themselves. They may also experience guilt when they first try to increase pleasant activities. Remind them that you are asking them to begin by setting very small, realistic goals. For instance, they can start by increasing one pleasant activity at a time. And, as mentioned earlier, some of these pleasant activities can be coupled with things they are already doing (habit stacking!), which will not cost any time or much effort. If they are still reluctant, you may incorporate some motivational strategies (MI) into this discussion (see Introduction).

Goal 5: Introduce the idea of tracking pleasant activities and mood to better understand the connection between the two

There is now an additional column on Worksheet 2.3: Looking at Connections: My Mood/Stress, Caregiving, and Activities, so parents can write down activities they did each day that influenced their mood. Given that parents are in the initial stage of understanding the connection between their activities and their mood, please hand them Worksheet 2.3 and instruct them to write down any activity that influenced their mood in either direction (more positive or more negative). As parents gain a better understanding of what "dials up" or "dials down" their mood, they can make changes to increase pleasant activities and to attempt to decrease activities that have a negative influence on their mood or that waste time they could better spend on activities that bring them more joy (e.g., spending an hour playing a game on their cell phone, scrolling through Instagram or Facebook).

Some parents might prefer to keep track of their activities on a calendar on their mobile phone (e.g., Google Calendar or iCal). In fact, the Google Calendar mobile application has a function that allows you to set goals in areas such as exercise, family/friends, me time, and organization—which is very fitting for the things we are asking parents to do. Keeping track of activities and progress toward goals on a mobile device has the added benefit of being portable and with the parent most of the time. Mobile phones also allow us to set alarm reminders to track activities or do a scheduled activity.

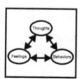

Encourage parents to take a "curious stance" as they investigate the connection between their activities and mood. A curious stance is helpful because it is natural for automatic judgments or criticisms of themselves or others to arise during this process. Remind parents that, over the course of treatment, you will be working on all parts of the CBT model, including thoughts. For now, they are taking an initial positive step toward better understanding the connection between activities (i.e., their behaviors) and their mood (i.e., feelings) so that they can work to increase the types of pleasant activities that have the greatest influence on their own mood.

On Worksheet 2.3: Looking at Connections: My Mood/Stress, Caregiving, and Activities, there is an additional column for monitoring your activities. When you do a pleasant activity that you identified today, make sure to write that down in this column. You can also write other activities in this column that had either a negative or positive effect on your mood each day. You can put a plus symbol next to the activities that had a positive influence on your mood.

Some people prefer to do their activity monitoring on a mobile device instead of using paper forms, which is perfectly fine and may be much easier because you usually have your mobile phone with you. You can also set alarms to remind you to write down what you are doing and how you are feeling. [If they prefer this, ask parents if they already have a way to monitor activities electronically or provide suggestions like the Google Calendar mobile application. See Module 3 for guidance on working with a calendar system.]

Your mood monitoring will be important to the success you will have in changing how you feel by changing what you do. [Refer to the CBT model again if needed.] *Time is unfortunately limited for most parents so you will want to focus on increasing those activities that have the greatest positive impact on your mood, which differs for everyone. By monitoring and observing connections between your activities and mood, you will learn what those activities are for you!*

Also, as you take this step towards better understanding the connection between your activities and your mood, you may notice that you have negative judgments about yourself or others. Try to be curious about the connections between your activities and mood, and know that we will address negative thinking later in the program. Remember, it is easiest to change what we do (our behavior) to influence how we think and feel!

Home Practice

At the end of the session, give the parent the Parent Summary and Handout 2.1: Special Time Guidelines if they have not received them yet. When you assign home practice to the parent, it is a good time to check in with them to see if they have any questions.

Home practice for this module includes:

- Completing Worksheet 2.1: Special Time Record Form
- Completing Worksheet 2.3: Looking at Connections: My Mood/ Stress, Caregiving, and Activities

Module 3: Maintaining a Consistent Schedule and Time Management

(Recommended Length: 1 or 2 Sessions)

Materials Needed for the Module

Forms, parent summaries, worksheets, and handouts appear in Appendix A: Client Materials, located at the end of this therapist guide. You may photocopy this material for your clients, or you may download these items from the Treatments ThatWork web site at www.oxfordclinicalpsych. com/ADHDparenting. For a therapist outline of this and all modules, go to Appendix B: Therapist Outlines.

Parent Materials

- Module 3 Parent Summary
- Worksheet 3.1: Categorizing Tasks
- Worksheet 3.2: Looking at Connections: My Mood/Stress, Caregiving, and Activities
- Worksheet 3.3: Special Time Record Form
- Handout 3.1: Sample Routines

Assessment to Be Given at Every Session

- Form B: Top Problems

Given the importance of home practice, it is critical to take a few minutes to review parents' practice since the last session. Taking time for this review each week not only conveys the importance of home practice but also helps to troubleshoot any problems they encountered before covering new material. Note that this home practice review can be done in either individual or group formats.

Module 2 taught parents about the importance of increasing pleasant activities with their child (Special Time) and on their own (identifying specific activities that are important to them and can be added to their schedule). Review Worksheet 2.1: Special Time Record Form, Worksheet 2.2: Pleasant Activities, and Worksheet 2.3: Looking at Connections: My Mood/Stress, Caregiving, and Activities. If parents did not practice at home, spend time reviewing the rationale for home practice and help them to troubleshoot any problems they encountered. If needed, you can bring in MI to motivate behavior change (see Introduction). You can use some of the following questions to facilitate the home practice review:

Special Time

- *Were you able to practice Special Time last week? What activities did your child choose? What was your child's reaction?*
- *How did you feel during Special Time? (Was it hard to relax? Did your mood change?)*
- *How did it go avoiding questions and directing? Did any challenges come up?*

Monitoring Mood and Pleasant Activities

- *Have you been monitoring your mood? Are you having any difficulty with this—remembering to do it, coming up with the mood rating, and so on?*
- *What pleasant activities did you do since we last met? Any trouble with this that I can help you with?*

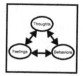

If needed, review what was discussed in Module 1 with Special Time as an example of a pleasant activity that can have a positive influence on the parent's mood (draw the cognitive-behavioral therapy [CBT] triangle and arrow pointing from behavior to feelings to review this concept). If parents mention having unpleasant feelings during Special Time, refer to the CBT model and ask if they were aware of thoughts about themselves, their child, or parenting during Special Time.

Therapist Note

Make sure to adjust the home practice review based on what was assigned in the previous session. If topics haven't been covered yet, omit the questions about that content from the home practice review. Also, if this home practice review does not include content that has been covered and assigned for home practice (e.g., if you are doing modules in a different order), make sure to expand the home practice review to include all assigned items.

Overall Module 3 Goals and Rationale

During Module 3, parents learn to develop and maintain a consistent household schedule and daily routines, both with their child and for themselves. This involves learning to use a *prioritized task list* if they don't already do so.

All children benefit from consistent structure and routines, but children with attention-deficit/hyperactivity disorder (ADHD) can be especially reactive when their environment is unpredictable or chaotic (think, orchid!). External structure can scaffold the child with ADHD's own sense of organization. In other words, if children themselves feel internally disorganized, the adults around them can provide a sense of external structure and organization. Thus, being planful about how to structure the family's daily routines (e.g., doing homework before the child is too tired and/or their ADHD medication has worn off), breaking down morning and bedtime routines into clear and manageable steps (e.g., brush teeth, change into pajamas, read for 10 minutes), and making sure the child gets adequate sleep will help to prevent child misbehavior and make it more likely that the child with ADHD will more easily follow through with the steps of their daily routines. Repeating routines consistently over the long term makes these routines automatic, ultimately reducing parent–child conflict.

In many families, parents of children with ADHD struggle with executive function or attention difficulties themselves. Teaching parents to implement a consistent daily schedule and to more effectively manage their time also serves to reduce parental stress and frustration, which can contribute to harsh or negative parenting and the negative sequelae of a dysregulated parent and poor parent–child relationship. Teaching parents to impose more structure onto their daily lives will also help them to be proactive versus reactive in their parenting. With your support, parents can think about other areas of their lives where routines can be helpful (e.g., reviewing and prioritizing a task list for the next day before they leave work so they may arrive home with less stress, hanging their keys on the same hook when they walk into the house, going to bed on time to get adequate sleep, etc.). An organized parent is going to be much better able to help their child with ADHD be organized and on top of things—and to do so more calmly! In this module, you will work with parents on the basics of scheduling and time management so that their households will run more smoothly and their children with ADHD will know what to expect. The ultimate goal, with practice, is for the child to be on "autopilot" when moving through the many steps of the morning, homework, or bedtime routines. This can lead to a more organized and harmonious household.

Specific goals for this module include

- **Goal 1:** Teach parents about the importance of maintaining a consistent and predictable daily schedule for the child with ADHD and the family as a whole.
- **Goal 2:** Work with the parent to thoughtfully schedule daily activities, such as sleep and wake times, mealtimes, and homework time to optimize the child's success.
- **Goal 3:** Work with the parent on developing consistent daily routines (e.g., breaking down the morning and evening routines into component parts).
- **Goal 4:** Introduce time management strategies (e.g., a prioritized to-do list) to help parents more effectively scaffold and model time management for their child with ADHD.

■ **Goal 5:** Help parents understand the value of consistent household structure while remaining *flexible* in the face of unexpected changes to help with their own and their child's emotion regulation.

Module 3 Content (Divided by Goals)

Goal 1: Teach parents about the importance of maintaining a consistent and predictable daily schedule for the child with ADHD and the family as a whole

 Children with ADHD are more sensitive to their environments and tend to thrive on external structure and consistency given their own internal disorganization and difficulty maintaining attention. For all of the reasons outlined in the previous section, maintaining a consistent and predictable daily schedule for the child and family is an important "antecedent" that can improve the happiness and functioning of the entire family. In other words, if the child lacks internal structure and organization, parental scaffolding and structure can create an external sense of organization, structure, and predictability for the child.

You can say something like,

All children thrive with external structure, and children with ADHD are even more sensitive to the negative effects of inconsistent schedules and the stress of having essential tasks not done when needed (especially when parents need to have more time and energy to keep their child on track!). A therapeutic environment for children with ADHD is one in which routines and necessary tasks are clear and predictable. How is your family doing now with establishing consistent routines and completing necessary tasks?

Goal 2: Work with the parent to thoughtfully schedule daily activities, such as sleep and wake times, mealtimes, and homework time to optimize the child's success.

 Begin this part of the session by brainstorming with the parent their day-to-day tasks and activities (alone and with the child). Such tasks usually include waking up, getting ready for school/work, daytime tasks/responsibilities (work, caring for house and children, etc.), getting ready for and attending extracurricular activities, mealtimes, homework, and bedtime. A good general principle to apply throughout the discussion of routines is that we often underestimate the time it takes to do something. For example, people can be regularly late for activities because they "get ready" to leave the house at the time they need to actually be leaving! The act of "leaving" (actually beginning to walk or drive away) can take up to 10 (or more) minutes. Thus, if this time is not included in the schedule, one will always be late! This proactive, planful thought process will make daily routines go more smoothly.

Sleep

Sleep is absolutely critical for children with ADHD and their parents! If you ask parents to remember back to when their child was an infant, they will likely remember the "mental fog" they felt when they were waking up several times per night to feed and change the baby. We know that many individuals with ADHD have more difficulty sleeping (which can sometimes be exacerbated by stimulant medication), and they are also more sensitive to "sleep debt" than the average person. Lack of sleep can affect mood, executive functioning, and overall health for everyone—making everything worse. Similarly, parents will be more irritable, less patient, and less effective when they are themselves sleep-deprived (as so many parents are these days). For all of these reasons, the best place to start when arriving at a daily schedule is to begin with ensuring that the child and parent are getting adequate sleep.

Refer to the American Academy of Pediatrics (AAP) sleep guidelines (see Box 3.1) to help facilitate the discussion of the family's sleep schedule and the factors that contribute to insufficient sleep time. Working backward from the AAP guidelines on the amount of sleep needed at various ages, work with the parent to determine a consistent wake time and bedtime for the child. Help the parent consider what time the child has to leave for school/daycare and how long it generally takes them to get ready through the morning and evening routines. Ideally, this bedtime will be adhered to 7 days per week (i.e., including weekends) to reduce sleep debt and enhance the consistency of the routine.

Reducing Morning Stress

You may recommend that parents consider an earlier wake up time if they currently get themselves ready for the day while their child(ren) are awake. Getting up earlier reduces the demands for multitasking, and parents can focus on helping the child stay on track without the stress and distraction of getting themselves ready as well. Note that this will require the parents to go to bed a little earlier, too. Waking up a little bit earlier can also allow parents time for self-care (e.g., taking a shower, enjoying a cup of coffee, exercising, reading the news) that will put them in a better mental space to work effectively and calmly with their child(ren) during the morning routine.

Another strategy to make mornings less hectic (an antecedent) is for the parent and child to determine which tasks can be done the night before. For example, getting the child into a routine of packing their backpack as soon as homework is completed reduces the child's risk for misplacing the homework and/or forgetting to bring homework back to school, and it is one less thing to remember in the morning. Similarly, lunches can often be made the night before to ease the stress of the morning rush. Choosing clothes the night before can prevent stress about this decision in the morning. Depending on the child's age/developmental level, they can be involved in these tasks because they will need to learn to independently complete such routines as they grow older.

Meals

It is helpful to consider schedules for eating as well. Hunger can be an antecedent to misbehavior (kids and parents can get "hangry"), and acting proactively to ensure that snacks and meals are predictable and available can help to prevent problems. When working on the meal schedule, consider any appetite suppression the child experiences related to stimulant medication. It is important that the child eats a high-protein meal before taking medication and when they have an appetite later in the day to avoid the potential growth suppression effects of stimulant medication. To avoid side effects of insomnia, the medication must be given on a consistent schedule (if the child takes it too late it will interfere with sleep), and thus medication times and meals need to be planned carefully.

There are many benefits to shared family meals, including healthier eating habits, better psychological well-being, and even lower risk of substance use and delinquency for teens (Musick & Meier, 2012). Identifying a time in the schedule when families can share a meal together (usually dinner) is therefore worth the effort, and this is another situation where proactive planning can make a big impact on stress. Scheduling time for meal planning and preparation (you can even suggest that the parent add these tasks to the schedule they are developing during this session) can make it much easier to eat family meals on a tight time schedule during the week. This is also a time when parental expectations (i.e., thoughts) can be identified if they lead to increased stress. Giving themselves permission to prepare simple and fast meals and to reduce accommodation for picky eating (instead of making multiple different meals) can help the parent gain some needed time in their schedule.

It can be difficult for all family members to sit down and eat at the same time each day, but with some creativity and persistence families can often find some time in their schedule where this is possible. Examples include family breakfast (some days this is easier than dinner, with work schedules, school events, and extracurricular activities), sitting when the kids have an afternoon snack or dinner even if parents aren't eating at the same time (rather than using this time to get other chores done or have kids watch a screen while eating), or a ritual for a weekend meal (pancake breakfast on Saturdays, taco dinner on Tuesdays, pizza night on Fridays etc.). If you ask parents to share memories from their own childhood, they are likely to remember rituals like family dinners that were special because they were done consistently and they could count on them happening.

Homework

Homework is often a struggle for children with ADHD, so it is critical that homework is consistently done at a time that maximizes the child's attentional capacity. For example, if the child does not begin homework until they are tired from a long day, that fatigue will negatively impact their attention and mood, thereby exacerbating ADHD-related homework problems and parent–child conflict. Homework should also be done in a quiet room with few distractions (e.g., no TV, little noise from others).

Another factor to consider for children taking ADHD medications is that homework needs to be done when medication is active. Parents should work with their prescriber to understand the duration of action for their child's medication, which does vary somewhat by individual. For this reason, parents should observe and ask the child about their focus and ability to persist on tasks. This may require some experimentation with homework times over a few weeks.

Some parents report that their child needs a break after focusing all day at school, and this is a valid point. A snack and a brief rest after school is helpful for many children. However, caution the parents to not allow the child to engage in any activities (e.g., TV or video games) which can create a challenging transition. This is another situation where paying attention to antecedents is helpful—putting less desirable activities (homework, getting dressed) before more desirable activities (screens, toys) in the schedule can prevent misbehavior that occurs when kids have to leave a desired activity to do something less desirable. Putting things in the schedule *in the right order* helps to maximize child attention and cooperation. Breaks can be a helpful antecedent, but parents need to make sure the break is rejuvenating and doesn't interfere with task completion.

The timing of activities like homework in your child's schedule is important. Children will naturally choose to do more desirable activities first, and parents then have challenges with transitions and the child's ability to focus on necessary tasks like homework. Children will sometimes say they need a break, and it is true that too many "have-to's" in your child's schedule will decrease motivation! However, the order in which things are done and choosing break times and activities that are rejuvenating (versus those that create conflict) must be considered when planning your child's schedule.

Help parents understand that, in general, a "when-then" approach is often most effective ("*when* you finish your homework, *then* you can go outside to play/have screen time"). This can also have the long-term effect of teaching children to delay gratification, get the essential tasks done first, and then reward themselves with a more preferred activity and deserved break. You can note that this strategy works for parents as well, and many adults benefit at home and work from using the *Premack principle*: a behavior that happens reliably (more desirable behavior) can be used as a reinforcer for a behavior that occurs less reliably (less desirable behavior). You can ask parents how this principle might help them with tasks related to the schedule changes you've discussed today.

Children with ADHD often need support getting started, persisting, and/or completing tasks during homework. Talk with parents about skills that children need to complete homework (such as creating a to-do list, breaking larger tasks into smaller parts, estimating time needed to complete tasks, organizing materials, and designating a quiet work area) and how their child can be supported as they learn and develop these skills. Parenting skills reviewed throughout this therapist guide can also be applied to homework time. For example, parents should provide labeled praise (see Module 4) for getting started on homework, staying on task, working carefully, and putting completed homework in their folder). Parents can also actively ignore (see Module 5) complaining, tapping pencils, humming, or standing at the homework desk/table.

Bedtime

Bedtime is another challenging time because children rarely want to go to bed and miss all the fun! Parents should estimate the time it takes for the child to get ready for bed and even allow for some extra time given that things usually take longer than expected. Remind the parent that we often underestimate the time it takes to do something if we include the time needed for preparation and transitions. Sleep routines (including reading together) are essential for good sleep hygiene. Screens, on the other hand, can have a negative impact on sleep quality and should be avoided for 30–120 minutes before bedtime. (If relevant, refer to the Resources section at the end of this module for links with more information for parents about the effects of screen time on sleep.) For older children who may have their own mobile devices, these should be removed from the bedroom to avoid screen time after the parent leaves the room. There are also ways for parents to monitor and turn off devices remotely to limit conflict around screen time limits (see Resources). It can be beneficial to have the goal of everyone in the family following a calming routine in the hour before the children's bedtime to put the whole house in "sleep mode," taking the noise level and even the lights down a notch to prepare the child for bed.

Special Time and Pleasant Activities

Special Time (see Module 2) should be added to the daily schedule to increase the likelihood that it will happen each day. Thoughtfully consider with the parent how much time is possible (ideally 10 minutes) and the natural time of day this could most easily fit into the schedule (e.g., after dinner or at bedtime). The goal is to do Special Time most days of the week, although it may be truncated on nights when the child has an extracurricular activity, or it can be folded into another activity like bath time, riding in the car (e.g., parent can allow the child to lead the conversation), or giving positive attention during an extracurricular activity.

Finally, when considering their own schedules, remind parents to include on the daily schedule their own pleasurable activities that are mood elevating, such as exercise, calling a friend/family member, reading a book, or watching a favorite TV show/Netflix episode. If parents seem overwhelmed, preview that you will soon talk about ways to approach and prioritize tasks to help them protect time for self-care activities. You can also validate that, during certain parenting "seasons," it is more difficult to practice self-care and that is why you will support them in finding ways to move in the right direction—it doesn't have to be a perfect schedule, just one that considers parent needs and mental/physical health.

As parents write their schedule, if there are busy days with little unstructured time for the parents' own pleasurable activity and Special Time, they can try to identify a short time where the parent and child can engage in a pleasurable activity together like doing a short yoga practice together at home (there are many free yoga videos online), watching a favorite TV show together, or playing a game of cards.

Additional Considerations

Children with ADHD benefit from spending time outdoors and engaging in physical activity (e.g., Gawrilow, Stadler, Langguth, Naumann, & Boeck, 2016). That can often be challenging to fit in, especially when the weather is not optimal for outdoor activities. If physical activity has not come up during the discussion of daily routines, ask about it and help parents think about where they can fit it in. It can be as simple as taking a walk after dinner, doing yoga together (may double as a parent pleasant activity), going for a bike ride, having a "dance party," or running around the house!

Also, parents and children often have weekly activities that may change the daily schedule. This may include doctor's appointments, sports, religious activities, or irregular parent work schedules. Think ahead with parents about how these activities may impact the daily routine and how to keep the daily routine as consistent and predictable as possible. Discuss with parents the benefits of previewing changes to the routine with their child as a helpful antecedent and learning opportunity for their child. In addition, encourage parents to think about the things that may get in the way of them maintaining their schedule and plan ahead for those things, too. For example, parents can put their mobile phones away if they think they may be interrupted during an activity chosen for relaxation. A theme here is to help parents be proactive (as opposed to reactive) in anticipating and planning for deviations from the daily schedule.

> **Goal 3: Work with the parent on developing consistent daily routines (e.g., breaking down the morning and evening routines into component parts)**

Each daily routine we have discussed thus far is actually a complex organizational task with multiple steps. Multistep routines or activities tax the attentional capacity of most children with ADHD (as well as parents who struggle with their own executive functioning deficits). Have the parent walk through the steps of their or their child's morning routine: wake up, shower, brush/floss teeth, eat breakfast, get dressed, get backpack ready (ideally done the night before), get shoes (and coat) on, and get out the door (more or less!). Homework involves writing down the assignment, bringing home necessary materials, getting started, reading directions, completing the homework, checking one's work, and putting it back in a folder and then in the backpack (not to mention remembering to turn it in!). That means homework consists of eight steps. This type of complex organizational task taps exactly the distractibility, forgetfulness, and disorganization that characterize ADHD. This is greatly compounded when caregivers themselves also struggle with attention/executive functioning difficulties.

Breaking down these complex, multistep routines is a challenging but essential skill for children with ADHD to learn, especially as they move toward greater independence in middle school, high school, and eventually college or other postsecondary settings. Working with the parent and child together (if the child can be present in session, or coaching the parent to work with the child later at home if the child is not present) is an important exercise.

We usually recommend beginning with *one daily routine at a time* (additional routines can be added after the family experiences success with the first one). Attacking all routines at once may be overwhelming for the parent, and success with the first routine can motivate and give the parent the confidence to add others. Brainstorming together, it is useful to create a step-by-step checklist that can be written on a whiteboard (dry-erase board) or printed on a paper/poster board that is hung prominently in the home. Give parents Handout 3.1, Sample Routines, and review it with them. This handout provides a good example of daily routines for a school-aged child, and you can talk with parents about how it would look different for a younger child. For example, pictures (rather than words) are helpful for younger children who cannot yet read. Involving the child in this process of breaking down and writing out steps (or finding the pictures) gives them more ownership of their routine. The child may write out the routine in their own words or decorate the poster with their favorite things. Then, as each step is completed, the child can check it off and move on to the next step.

Note that this is a good time to remind parents to praise the child for staying on task and completing each step of the routine (see Module 4 for more detail on this). Some parents are resistant to doing this because they may feel that the child *should* be doing these things on their own without praise; however, you can gently remind such parents that their child is *currently* not doing these things independently, and doing so requires more effort from the child than things they have mastered (or for peers of the same age without ADHD). You may also remind parents that ADHD is a brain-based disorder that makes it harder for their child to focus, and more frequent praise for each step of the routine is part of providing a therapeutic environment for their child.

Children may also receive a reward/reinforcer for completing their routine in a timely manner, such as a special treat with their lunch or the natural reinforcer of some time to watch TV or play on a tablet before they head out the door (although, as noted earlier, disengaging the child from these activities may become an issue, in which case this should be avoided). You can let parents know that, later in the program, you will discuss more structured ways of rewarding their child to motivate them during challenging times of day (Module 10). For now, try to help parents consistently use the skills suggested in this module to see if this resolves the struggle.

> *Goal 4: Introduce time management strategies (e.g., a prioritized to-do list) to help parents more effectively scaffold and model time management for their child with ADHD*

Managing a schedule and getting things done may not be an issue for every parent with whom you work, but for some parents who struggle with their own motivation, procrastination, or attention problems, scheduling and accomplishing goals is a major challenge. This is especially true for parents who suffer from depression or adult ADHD.

Therapist Note

Some parents participating in this program may have told you at this point that they have a mental health disorder. That may be why they selected this program. Other parents may not have reported a mental health diagnosis, but you may suspect one. If a parent is experiencing mental health difficulties that require more than what is provided in this program, this could be a good time to gently provide referrals for an evaluation, medication (e.g., in the case of undiagnosed adult ADHD), or their own therapy.

 All of the strategies discussed in this module involve *scheduling*. Parents have so many things going on in their day-to-day lives that it is nearly impossible for someone to remember everything without some type of calendar system. Some parents may carry a planner book or use an online calendar already (like Google Calendar or Tasks), but others will not be using such tools and will need more support with this.

Calendar Systems

If parents are already using a calendar system, take some time to learn about their system, how well it is working, and difficulties they experience. Troubleshoot with them any pitfalls of their current system, and ask if they are interested in your suggestions to help with scheduling (using motivational interviewing [MI] style). Common issues are that parents have a calendar but forget to check it (or forget to add items to it), have multiple calendars (which can be very confusing and result in double booking), or are simply inconsistent in using the system.

Online calendar systems are ideal because they are with us all the time (given that most people use smartphones) and they allow us to enter recurrent activities and set alarms to remind us when to leave, etc. These online calendars can be shared with the co-parent, babysitter, or even with older children who have their own devices. Again, by using these strategies and incorporating the child in the process, the parent is teaching the child critical life skills that they can adopt on their own as they get older.

As you are working through the daily schedule, spend some session time entering the daily routine you worked out together into the parent's calendar system and set reminders. (You can often set multiple reminders, for example 15, 10, and 5 minutes before an activity.) Remind parents that previous skills/strategies learned in the program should be added to the calendar, including Special Time with the child and the parent's own pleasant activities (Module 2). Prepare the parent by setting the expectation that most systems for scheduling need some adjustments and to consider this a trial period when they will get good information to identify what works for them and what doesn't.

Prioritized To-Do Lists

With all of the competing demands on parents, it can be hard to keep track of everything they have to do. Also, there is not enough time in the day for parents to do all of these things! That is why keeping to-do lists and prioritizing tasks is such an important skill (and another skill that is useful to teach and model for the child). Many of the online calendar systems and scheduling apps have corresponding to-do lists that include an option to put in a deadline (e.g., Google Calendar and Tasks).

Many parents relate to the idea that too much time is spent on distracting (or delayable) tasks rather than having true priorities determine where our time goes. This is natural! However, many parents feel overwhelmed and guilty with thoughts of never doing enough. The *Eisenhower Matrix* (also known as the *Urgent-Important Matrix*) can be used to help parents view tasks based on their importance and urgency. This matrix stems from a quote by President Eisenhower: "I have two kinds of problems, the urgent and the important. The urgent are not important, and the important are never urgent." Tasks can be sorted into four quadrants—important and urgent, important and not urgent, urgent and not important, and not urgent and not important—that help us make decisions about how to spend our time. Give parents Worksheet 3.1: Categorizing Tasks, located in Appendix A, to complete as an in-session activity during this discussion.

Examples of the Urgent-Important Matrix include

- *Important and Urgent*: Comforting your child when they are hurt (do this right away)
- *Important and Not Urgent*: Teaching your child something (can be added to the schedule)
- *Urgent and Not Important*: Going to the store because you are out of milk (can be delegated if you don't have time or delayed)
- *Not Urgent and Not Important*: Making the bed (can be left undone)

Most parents find that there are not enough hours in the day to get everything done! When parenting a child with ADHD, your ability to effectively manage your time and energy is especially important given your child's needs for more support compared to their same-age peers. To reduce stress and increase feelings of accomplishment, using a system like the Eisenhower Matrix can help you to determine which tasks are most important for your family and which tasks may be distracting or able to be delayed. As you think about your daily schedule and the things we discussed today, can you think of any tasks/activities that get in the way of your priorities?

[Examples: If calls or emails are distracting, some parents find it helpful to put their phone away during certain parts of the routine (e.g., from 6 to 8 PM or 7 to 8 AM). If parents are very stressed about getting chores done when their child needs their support, seeing the task as delayable (or able to be delegated) can help parents prioritize what is most important in that moment.]

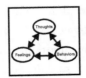

Indeed, parents may need to learn to *accept* that not all tasks will be completed each day and to be kind to themselves about the things that do not get done. They may need to adjust their standards (e.g., giving themselves permission to have a messy family room or to order take-out once in a while) or call in supports (co-parent, neighbor, babysitter, or cleaning person) if possible to get everything done with less stress. For a parent who has rigid thinking about expectations for themselves and their family ("I should be able to do this without help"), use the CBT model (thoughts-feelings-behaviors) to help them identify more helpful thinking to change how they feel. Module 4 gives more specific ways to help parents with changing their thinking, including their expectations of themselves and others that lead to feelings of stress, resentment, or anxiety.

Assertiveness (Saying "No" and Feeling OK About It)

For some parents, assertiveness skills (taught and practiced in Module 6) will need to be used so they do not overcommit and take on too many obligations. You can normalize that many people need practice to say "no" when they have the desire to help others and contribute. Being mindful of the *limits* of our energy and time can help us to make the commitments that are most important and to say "no" or "not at this time" when we need to. If this is particularly difficult for a parent, suggest a small step toward having more boundaries that can help with stress: have the parent practice saying, "I'll need to get back to you" when a request is made to give them additional time to decide if they can/want to add something to their to-do list and schedule. Adding a "pause" or waiting 24 hours before agreeing to something is a good rule of thumb. Co-parents may also need to think about the current division of responsibilities and changes that can help with times of day that are most stressful for the family. For example, sharing or delegating a task to a co-parent can make the morning or evening routines more manageable for both parents.

Maintaining enough energy to support your child and your own self-care will require saying "no" to requests and not doing things even though you would like to do them if time and energy were limitless. We will talk later in the program about assertiveness skills that can also help with managing your time and delegating. For this week, is there any boundary you can set (even a small one) that can protect you from taking on too much?

Goal 5: Help parents understand the value of consistent household structure while remaining flexible with unexpected changes to help with their own and their child's emotion regulation

Schedules, routines, and prioritized to-do lists are extremely helpful when they are approached with the *flexibility* needed for the realities of day-to-day life with children. When parents are too rigid, they are less likely to use good problem-solving skills and model good flexibility for their child.

You can ask, "*What things may influence your family's ability to follow a schedule or complete 'to do's' on any given day?*" Examples include illness, a co-parent traveling, a new activity starting, a large project due, and visitors.

Parents and children alike may have difficulty when there are changes to the schedule (especially if these changes are last-minute). Understanding that changes/challenges *will* occur in life and that *not everything is in our control* can help us calmly and strategically problem-solve when these things do happen. It helps to understand one's priorities (e.g., sleep, homework) and to consider what is *not* absolutely necessary to achieve on any given day (tidying up or other household chores). Sometimes dinner will need to be later (or frozen) to adjust to these changes, and that is OK! Remember, a calm and well-grounded parent helps the child to stay well-regulated.

In addition, schedules may need to change as activities are added or as children's needs change over time. Let parents know that if the schedule or routine isn't working at a later point, they should review the routine and make course corrections as needed.

Group Options: Here are a few questions to jump-start group discussion:

- *Can a few people share what has worked for them in terms of a daily schedule for your child/family? What has worked and not worked?*
- *What type of calendar system do you use and why do you like it?*
- *Does anyone use particular apps for a prioritized to-do list?*

Home Practice

At the end of each session, distribute the Parent Module Summary and reinforce the fact that the information discussed today will now be practiced at home. Home practice for this module includes:

- Implementing a daily schedule or routine
- Practicing using at least one of the time management techniques discussed in this session
- Completing Worksheet 3.2: Looking at Connections: My Mood/ Stress, Caregiving, and Activities
- Completing Worksheet 3.3: Special Time Record Form

Remind parents about the schedule/routine that you worked on in session and encourage them to test it out before the next session. Also, ask parents to identify one time management strategy they would like to try this week that they are not currently using (a calendar system, a prioritized to-do list, delegating or not doing a task that is not a priority, saying "I'll have to get back to you" or "Not at this time" to a request for something that will take time and is not a priority, etc.). Ask parents if they anticipate any problems with the home practice this week and troubleshoot.

> **Therapist Note**
>
> When presenting the two worksheets for home practice, parents may need you to explain why they need to do those home practices again this week. Although these skills were not discussed much in Module 3, practicing them until they become routine is essential to the success of this program. As parents incorporate pleasant activities and Special Time into their schedule, they will see a more positive mood and improved child behavior. If parents reported feeling better over the past week or noticed an improvement in their child's behavior, remind them of that and link it to their home practice completion. If they stop doing these things, they will not experience the full benefits of the program.

Resources

- Sleep
  https://www.aap.org/en-us/about-the-aap/aap-press-room/Pages/American-Academy-of-Pediatrics-Supports-Childhood-Sleep-Guidelines.aspx

- Screens

  https://www.sleepfoundation.org/articles/why-electronics-may-stimulate-you-bed
  https://www.fosi.org/good-digital-parenting/
  https://meetcircle.com

- Calendars/Schedules

  https://calendar.google.com
  https://www.cozi.com/

CHAPTER 4

Module 4: Praise and Changing Your Thinking to Feel Better

(Recommended Length: 1 or 2 Sessions)

Materials Needed for the Module

Forms, parent summaries, worksheets, and handouts appear in Appendix A: Client Materials, located at the end of this therapist guide. You may photocopy this material for your clients, or you may download these items from the Treatments ThatWork web site at www.oxfordclinicalpsych.com/ ADHDparenting. For an outline of this and all modules, go to Appendix B: Therapist Outlines.

Parent Materials

- Index cards
- Rubber bands
- Module 4 Parent Summary
- Worksheet 4.1: Catch Your Child Being Good
- Worksheet 4.2: Practice Hot Thoughts and Thinking Errors
- Worksheet 4.3: Looking at Connections: My Mood/Stress, Caregiving, Activities, and Thoughts
- Worksheet 4.4: Special Time and Child Behavior Record Form
- Handout 4.1: Thinking Errors and Strategies for Increasing Helpful and Decreasing Unhelpful Thoughts

■ Form B: Top Problems

Home Practice Review from Module 3

In Module 3, you taught parents about the benefits of maintaining a consistent schedule and routines, how to create a schedule that works for their family, and time management skills, including a prioritized to-do list. If parents did not practice at home, spend time reviewing the rationale for the home practice and help them to troubleshoot any problems they encountered implementing the skills. Some parents will need a lot of support to make these changes. You can use some of the following questions to facilitate the home practice review:

■ *What adjustments did you make to your schedule after our last session?*

■ *What routine did you choose to break down into steps, and how did that go? What was your child's reaction? Did any challenges come up?*

■ *What time management strategy did you try? Did you make any modifications to your calendar system or to-do list? How did that go?*

If needed during the home practice review, provide reminders that having a daily schedule and daily routines is an "antecedent" that sets the child up for success throughout the day. (You can draw the ABC model [see Module 1] and review the impact of antecedents on the child behavior.)

In earlier modules, you also covered Special Time, mood monitoring, and scheduling pleasant activities. It is important to briefly review the forms (or their calendars) and check in with parents about how their practice is going with all skills covered so far.

■ *Have you been monitoring your mood and activities? Are you having any difficulty with this—remembering to do it, coming up with the mood rating, and so on?*

■ *What about Special Time practice? Any trouble with this that I can help you with?*

Make sure to adjust the home practice review based on what was assigned in the previous session. If topics haven't been covered yet, omit the questions about that content from the home practice review. Also, if this home practice review does not include content that has been covered and assigned for home practice (e.g., if you are doing modules in a different order), make sure to expand the home practice review to include all assigned items.

Overall Module 4 Goals and Rationale

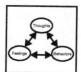

During Module 4, parents learn to praise their child to increase appropriate and desirable behaviors. They also learn that their own automatic thoughts about their child, parenting, and self can influence how they feel and behave. By learning specific common thinking errors and how to challenge them, parents develop an important skill that can help them with emotion regulation and improved mood, which can in turn affect their parenting. Parents will also be able to increase their sense of control by learning the thoughts-feelings-behaviors connection (refer to Module 2, where the cognitive-behavioral therapy [CBT] model was first introduced). If our reaction to situations is something we can change, then we will feel more capable and in control when challenging situations arise. In other words, although parents cannot always control a situation, they can learn to respond in new ways (in line with the CBT framework). Toward this end, specific strategies for increasing helpful and constructive thinking and decreasing negative or unhelpful thinking (particularly in relation to their parenting and child) will be taught in this module. As parents establish new ways of thinking, different feelings and actions will follow.

Specific goals for this module include

- **Goal 1:** Teach parents to praise their child's appropriate behavior and to use praise to increase "positive opposites" in order to influence their child's behavior.
- **Goal 2:** Teach parents the situations-thoughts-feelings connection to help them understand the relationship between automatic thoughts and feelings.

- **Goal 3:** Describe common thinking errors and practice how to challenge these errors in order to feel better.
- **Goal 4:** Teach ways to increase helpful thinking and reduce unhelpful thinking.

Module 4 Content (Divided by Goals)

> *Goal 1: Teach parents to praise their child's appropriate behavior and to use praise to increase "positive opposites" in order to influence their child's behavior*

Parental attention is very motivating for children, even if the parent's interactions with their child are generally more negative than positive. It is easy for children to learn that misbehaving is an effective way to get undivided attention from parents and teachers. This is especially true for behaviors that are attention-seeking, like whining, crying, or interrupting. That is why these are sometimes called "attention-seeking behaviors." These behaviors continue and grow when you pay attention to them. For example, when a child is in the classroom, they get 1/25th of the teacher's attention. But, when that child misbehaves, the teacher turns all their attention to the child who is misbehaving. Children may frequently gain adult attention this way. Sometimes parents, just like teachers, get in the habit of *not* giving attention to positive child behaviors and give more attention to negative behaviors. Parents and teachers may think they should just "let sleeping dogs lie," but instead, in this module and throughout this program, we will be working with parents to actively notice and praise the child's positive behaviors.

To begin this discussion, draw the ABC model on a whiteboard or paper (refer to Figure 4.1), and explain that what often happens naturally is that (1) negative behaviors are paired with attention from adults (which is a positive consequence) and (2) positive behaviors are paired with no attention/ignoring (which is a negative consequence). Make sure that parents understand that attention does not have to be positive for it to reinforce behaviors for children. Any attention is better than no attention!

Of course, parents do not intend to ignore their child's positive behaviors, but this is a common trap to fall into. It is important to normalize this

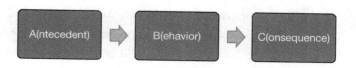

Figure 4.1

The ABC model.

for parents (you don't want them to feel bad!), but also emphasize that you will be working together to change this pattern.

Therapist Note

Some parents may benefit from learning more about the function of attention-seeking behaviors so that they can think more positively about their child. When children do attention-seeking behaviors, they are not being manipulative or "choosing" to bother their parents. Instead, these behaviors often have a history of "working" to engage others (consequence) and so they are likely to keep happening. That is why it is important for parents to actively try to notice when the child demonstrates appropriate behavior, especially when they are upset or are learning a new skill.

We want to change these pairings (i.e., negative behavior with attention; positive behavior with no attention) to make sure we are "growing" the appropriate behaviors. If parents react only to negative behaviors and don't notice when their child *is* behaving, their parent-child interactions will become increasingly negative, and it will feel like the parent is mostly criticizing or correcting. Over time, this dynamic diminishes the parent-child relationship, which is an important foundation for all of the other skills included in this treatment program.

 On your drawing of the ABC model of child behavior, show that child appropriate behavior (behavior) and caregiver positive attention (consequence) should be paired. When parents do this, they are encouraging their children to behave appropriately in the future while also strengthening their relationship.

The parent has already made important changes with Special Time and pleasant activities. By giving more attention to their child's positive behavior throughout the day, the scale will be tipped in increasingly positive directions and leave both the parent and child feeling better. Such positive spirals (as opposed to negative spirals) can be created in interactions as both parent and child become more positive. In other words, both parent and child will think, feel, and behave more positively.

How to Praise Effectively

For parents to give their child more attention for positive behavior, they can focus on "catching their child being good." When the parent sees their child doing something (anything) good—such as following a direction, putting good effort into something (even for a brief time) like homework, or playing nicely with siblings or friends—the parent will *praise* the child.

Teach parents to be as specific as possible with their praise, *telling their child exactly what they did that the parent liked*. Specific (or labeled) praises allow children to know exactly what is appreciated, and parents will be more likely to see that exact behavior again. Examples of specific praises can be shared with the parent, such as, "I like the way you asked politely," "That was really nice of you to share your toy with your sister," and "You are doing a great job sticking with your homework." Explain to parents that more vague praise like "Good job!" are not as useful or meaningful because the child will not know *exactly* what behavior the parent liked. Specific praises also have a bigger impact on the ratio of positive feedback to corrective feedback. Parents would need to give a lot more vague praises to tip the scale to more positive interactions with their child.

An especially important time to practice giving specific praises and to catch the child being good is when children are told to do something. Many parents feel that not following directions (either because of inattention or noncompliance) is one of the biggest problems for their child. Not following directions causes children to have trouble getting along with teachers, caregivers, and their peers. Children often receive negative attention (yelling, nagging, arguing) when they don't listen to directions. It is therefore important for adults to not miss the chance to give children positive attention whenever they do listen. Instead of moving on, praise can be used to increase this behavior.

It is also important for parents to understand that children with attention and behavior problems have to *work harder* to do what is expected and deserve credit for this effort.

Some parents are reluctant to praise their child for things that should be done or for expected behaviors. In this case, you can review the information about how their child's attention-deficit/hyperactivity disorder (ADHD) impacts the ability to perform expected behaviors. Children are supported when they receive more frequent praise for effort and progress, rather than penalized for the challenges that arise due to inattention and/or impulsivity/hyperactivity.

Help parents to understand that their child doesn't have to do something *perfectly* or for a long period of time to praise them. It is important to (1) praise *effort* as well as success and (2) praise *progress* along the way. Such praise can motivate children to keep going when they are working on a less desirable, challenging, or frustrating task. Praising effort and progress can be especially helpful for behaviors that can be considered "positive opposites." Positive opposites are the appropriate behaviors that are the opposite of a child's challenging behaviors. For example:

- The positive opposite of yelling is playing quietly.
- The positive opposite of dawdling is getting started on something right away.
- The positive opposite of bossiness is compromising or going along with someone else's idea.
- The positive opposite of demanding behavior is staying calm and being flexible when something does not go as wanted or expected.

If parents begin to give specific praises for effort, progress, and the positive opposite of challenging behaviors, they will be using their attention in a powerful way. They will also train themselves to think more positively about their child(ren).

Therapist Note

Some parents may have concerns about praising their child and possible negative effects on child motivation and self-esteem. Genuine praise that focuses on effort and the child's approach to tasks is recommended and has been shown to have a positive effect on child behavior, self-esteem, and motivation. Praises that are insincere, inflated, or put too high standards on children (perfect, the best, comparing them to others) can be less effective.

Ask parents *"What are examples of behaviors you can praise this week?"* Encourage them to think of the positive opposites of problem behaviors. If rough play is a problem, praise any gentle behaviors, including efforts or progress that may not be perfect yet. On Worksheet 4.1: Catch Your Child Being Good, there is a section for parents to write in specific behaviors they want to praise their child for this week. Parents should also be sure to incorporate the specific praises during Special Time this week.

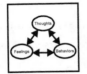 You can acknowledge that giving positive attention to your child is *harder when you are feeling down or stressed*, but remember, by acting in this positive way, parents may think and feel more positively and have a positive impact on their child's behavior.

> **Group Option:** Have the group generate ideas for specific behaviors that can be praised. You can prompt the group to think of the behaviors they would most like to see change in their children (top problems) and generate a list of positive opposites.

Therapist Note

Some parents of children with ADHD struggle with deep, ingrained patterns of negative thinking about themselves, others, and/or the world that may require individual CBT. These thought patterns can interfere with the parent's ability to see the positive aspects of the child's behavior or the progress the child is making. This may be especially true for parents with a history of recurrent depressive episodes, anger management issues, or trauma. Consider a referral for the parent if the CBT work in this program does not appear to be enough to address the parent's own interpersonal difficulties.

Culture can also impact a parent's beliefs about the appropriateness of praise and giving positive attention for expected behaviors. Spend time addressing concerns and identify who else may need to receive information about the intervention so that the parent(s) can feel supported by extended family and community members.

> *Goal 2: Teach parents the situation-thoughts-feelings connection to help them understand the relationship between automatic thoughts and feelings*

When parents have struggled with their child's challenging behaviors and impairment related to inattention and hyperactivity/impulsivity, parental patterns of thinking can develop that interfere with their ability to see the positive aspects of their child's behavior, such as effort and progress that has been made. The history of struggles can lead parents to a "cup-half-empty" mindset and automatic reactions that are more negative, global, and generalized. By helping parents to become aware of their automatic thoughts about their child, their parenting, and themselves, parents will have more success with specific parenting skills like praise.

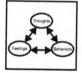

For this goal, start by reminding parents that there is a strong connection between how we *think* and how we *feel*. Difficult things happen; however, *what we tell ourselves about what happened* can influence how we feel. Challenging situations lead to automatic reactions including thoughts, but the good news is that even if we can't change a situation (it's already happened), we CAN change how we think about it. Refer back to Figure 2.1, if needed, and on the whiteboard draw the CBT model to illustrate this concept for the parent.

Now you can provide some examples of the range of situations that can elicit automatic thoughts that lead to unpleasant feelings. Examples include

- When the parent is criticized by someone (about their parenting, a decision they made)
- When parents don't feel appreciated by their family, children, or others
- When parents don't get credit for what they are doing (with children, at home, at work)
- When they don't meet their expectations for themselves in parenting and other situations (yelled at their child, forgot something important, feel like they aren't doing enough at home or work)
- When someone doesn't say or do something that the parent expected of them (their partner drops the ball or doesn't agree with them)
- Having things turn out differently than parents expected (their children's reaction to something, changes in their health, work, or friendships)

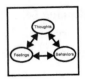

To help parents understand the relationship between situations, thoughts, and feelings even better, you can introduce Albert Ellis's *ABCD model* (not to be confused with the ABC model of child behavior discussed throughout this program!) to better understand our reactions to certain situations (see Figure 4.2). Often, people view the situation they are in as causing an emotion ("I felt frustrated because my child had a tantrum"); however, they do not consider that *what they tell themselves* (i.e., their thoughts or "self-talk") *about what happens* also contributes to how they feel. Ellis's ABCD method can help parents to better understand how they think about difficult situations in their life and how this leads to less healthy emotional functioning. It's not that unpleasant feelings go away, but the intensity of feelings and the degree of responsibility or control can change significantly. The theory is that feelings of being upset come more from what a person says to themselves about the situation than from the actual events.

Illustrate the model on a whiteboard to help parents follow along as you explain.

Most people assume that the Activating Event causes you to have an emotional reaction or Consequence, C. Rather it is what you believe or say to yourself about the Activating Event that causes the emotional reaction, C.

You can walk through an example, like getting negative feedback from someone about a parenting decision you made. Someone might notice thoughts and beliefs about this situation such as, "I never do the right thing" or "Everyone should agree with my decisions." These thoughts lead to strong emotions like feeling very down or angry.

- A = Activating Event
- B = Beliefs and Thoughts about the event
- C = Emotional Consequences
- D = Disputing or challenging thinking errors

Figure 4.2

The Ellis ABCD method.

Extreme thoughts are called *hot thoughts*. The parent can consider that, rather than the negative feedback (the situation) making them feel this way, it is also *their thinking in response to the negative feedback that leads to their feeling upset.*

Explain that in this same situation, if someone else had thoughts like, "It's okay for that person to disagree with me," "I made a good decision," or "I can be open and consider others' opinions," this way of thinking would lead to different emotions (such as feeling less stressed, calmer, or more confident).

Make sure to validate that many people feel disappointed or upset when challenging situations happen. Of course we can *wish or prefer* to have situations go a certain way, and unpleasant feelings are a part of life. However, when we have thoughts like "should" or "must," we can get stuck in strong and less healthy feelings. The thought "*I wish* that person agreed with me" leads to different feelings than the thought "That person *SHOULD or MUST* agree with me."

Now go through an example that relates to the parent's child displaying a challenging behavior. You can ask, *"What are some hot thoughts that occur when your child is having a tantrum or demanding something or not listening?"* [Note: Make sure this example is relevant to the child's top problems.]

Provide some examples if needed, such as: "My daughter never listens," "My son won't have any friends," "They are doing this to me on purpose," or "She makes everything harder than it should be." Validate that when our child is struggling, we can have automatic thoughts that make us very angry or worried (and often both). When kids struggle with following directions and rules, social skills, and managing strong feelings, we can change our thinking to more helpful thoughts. Ask the parent if they sometimes have thoughts that are more balanced when their child's behavior is challenging and provide some examples of helpful self-talk if needed: "We are working on this," "This is hard for my child right now," "Even adults have trouble staying calm when they have intense feelings," or "There are things I can do to help them deal with this challenge." These thoughts are more specific and time limited (rather than generalized and global).

Group Option: Ask group members to share thoughts they have in relation to their child and/or their parenting. Write these thoughts on the board. Then ask other group members to generate more helpful thoughts for each of these examples. Often it is easier for parents to challenge/reframe other people's thoughts than their own, but this can be an important first step in changing their own thinking.

Goal 3: Describe common thinking errors and practice how to challenge these errors in order to feel better

The beliefs or thoughts that cause parents to have more intense emotional reactions are also referred to as *thinking errors*. Thinking errors are automatic ways of thinking that are biased and lead to negative feelings. Specific thinking errors have been identified that lead to people feeling down and stressed/anxious. When people learn these thinking errors, they can notice when they happen and shift to more helpful thinking.

Use Handout 4.1: Thinking Errors and Strategies for Increasing Helpful and Decreasing Unhelpful Thoughts, located in Appendix A at the end of this therapist guide, to introduce four thinking errors common to parents that may occur for them in relation to their child, their parenting, and other situations.

Therapist Note

This module also describes six additional thinking errors. If you think the parent would benefit from learning about additional thinking errors or that certain thinking errors are particularly relevant for the parent, you can present some or all of them. We do not want to overwhelm parents with too much information! We recommend that all parents learn about the first four thinking errors, which are included on Handout 4.1 (shoulds, all-or-none, filtering, and labeling).

Our thoughts are automatic (kind of like breathing) so we may not notice that our automatic thoughts are biased or unhelpful. Another way of saying this is that we can have automatic "thinking errors," but we treat these thoughts as facts. Thoughts are not facts! When we are feeling stressed, anxious, or down, our automatic thoughts can become more negative and extreme, which leads to more upset feelings. Becoming more aware of our thoughts and our most common thinking errors allows us to catch them and challenge them. We are now going to talk about how to do this.

You can next describe the thinking errors and provide examples that are most relevant for the parent and family.

Thinking Errors

Shoulds

*The first thinking error is thinking in **SHOULDS**: When you have rules about how you or other people should or must act, this often leads to feeling guilty or self-critical ("I should _____ more,") and becoming angry with others when they don't follow your expectations ("Others must _____ ").*

For example:

- *My child should be able to get ready for school independently at their age!*
- *My spouse should be helping more with these household chores!*
- *I should be able to keep my house looking better than this!*
- *Everyone else's parents help with their grandchildren!*
- *Other moms balance everything so much more easily!*

Ask the parent to generate some of the "should thoughts" that they have:

These can be thoughts about yourself, your child, or your parenting.

Therapist Note

If a parent responds that a "should" thought is true, you can validate and use it as an opportunity to discuss the difference between a "true" or "real" thought and a helpful thought. A thought that includes "should" or "must" may be giving us important information about our values or changes that need to be made. However, helpful thoughts lead to helpful actions. *Ruminating* (having the same thought over and over) and getting stuck in "shoulds" leads to feeling upset, not feeling better or making a change. A "should" or "must" thought may also keep us from accepting a situation and the aspects of a situation that are out of our control.

All-or-None

> *The second common thinking error is ALL-OR-NONE THINKING.*
> *In all-or-nothing thinking, you think in absolutes like always, never,*
> *perfect, or terrible. When we are fighting with someone, we might*
> *think in extremes.*

For example:

- *My daughter never does what she is told!*
- *My son always puts up a fight when I tell him to do something!*
- *My child always wakes up in a bad mood.*
- *My spouse never helps with the kids.*
- *Other people's houses are always neater than mine.*
- *Other moms always look better than me.*

"Never" and "always" thoughts are rarely 100% true, and, by thinking this way, parents may feel worse and behave in ways that they may later regret.

Ask the parent to think of recent examples of "all-or-none" thoughts.

Filtering

> *A third thinking error is **FILTERING**: We filter out the OK*
> *or good things about a situation and we are left only with the*
> *negative aspects. The good things "don't count" and the negative*
> *things are magnified. For example, when someone asks how our*
> *day was and we say, "My day was awful" because my child got*
> *in trouble at school. We filtered out the fact that we had a good*
> *conversation with a friend, got something done on our to-do list,*
> *or that our child cleaned their room when asked. Your vision of*
> *reality becomes darkened like the drop of ink that discolors the*
> *entire beaker of water.*

For example:

- *I did not get a thing done today!*
- *My child had a terrible semester in school!*
- *That project was a complete failure!*

Ask the parent(s) if they notice this type of thinking when something negative happens.

Labeling

> *A fourth thinking error is **LABELING**. When we give labels to ourselves or someone else, we are discounting a lot of information. For example, after making a mistake, you think "I'm a loser" instead of "I made a mistake this time." Or you think "My child/ spouse is selfish" instead of "My child has a hard time sharing sometimes."*

For example:

- *My child is a lazy student.*
- *I am not a patient person.*
- *My child's teacher is insensitive.*
- *My child is a mean kid.*
- *My partner is selfish.*

Such thoughts can lead to angry or depressed feelings and behaviors. Ask the parent if they have recently thought in labels when thinking of themselves or others.

Therapist Note

Six additional thinking errors are described here. Reviewing ten thinking errors at once may be overwhelming for parents, so we recommend choosing and focusing on the thinking errors you view as most relevant for the parent.

Disqualifying the Positive

> *A fifth thinking error is **DISQUALIFYING THE POSITIVE**. You reject positive experiences by insisting that they "don't count" for some reason or other. In this way, you can maintain a negative belief that is contradicted by your everyday experiences.*

For example:

- *That was just lucky.*
- *That only happened because . . .*
- *I helped the kids with their homework, but the house is a mess and we had fast food for dinner.*
- *It must have been an easy exam if my child passed.*

Ask the parent if they notice a pattern of disqualifying the positive in certain situations, relationships, or areas like productivity.

Jumping to Conclusions

A sixth thinking error is JUMPING TO CONCLUSIONS. You make a negative interpretation even though there are no definite facts that convincingly support your conclusions.

For example:

- *The teacher called, so something must be wrong.*
- *If I forget to do something for tomorrow, others will be very upset with me.*
- *If I invite someone I don't know that well to a social activity, they will say no.*
- *No one will come to my child's birthday party.*

Ask the parent if they tend to jump to conclusions and assume a negative outcome will occur.

Catastrophizing

A seventh thinking error is CATASTROPHIZING. When we catastrophize, we overestimate the likelihood that the worst outcome will occur, which causes us to worry.

For example:

- *My child won't have friends (after receiving an email about an incident at school).*
- *I will lose my job (after making a mistake at work).*
- *Our relationship will end (after a conflict).*

Ask the parent if they notice thinking about "worst case" outcomes that results in feeling very anxious.

Mind Reading

*An eighth thinking error is **MIND READING**. You think that someone is reacting negatively to you and don't check out whether this is true or not.*

For example:

- *Others think I am a bad parent.*
- *The teacher thinks my child is. . . .*
- *My partner thinks I am. . . .*

Ask the parent if they automatically assume someone is thinking negatively of them when there is no evidence of this.

Emotional Reasoning

*A ninth thinking error is **EMOTIONAL REASONING**. You assume that your negative emotions necessarily reflect the way things are: "I feel it, therefore it must be true."*

Ask the parent if they assume their negative emotions are giving them accurate information.
For example:

- *I feel worried so something must be wrong.*
- *I feel guilty so I must have done something wrong.*

Personalization

*A tenth thinking error is **PERSONALIZATION**. You see yourself as the cause of some negative external event for which, in fact, you are not primarily responsible.*

For example:

- *My child's low grade is because I have not done enough.*
- *Others aren't happy because I didn't have a good plan for the day.*
- *My child is having a tantrum because of what I did (e.g., taking something away).*

Ask the parent if they take responsibility for how others are feeling or for how situations turn out even though there are many things out of their control.

After presenting all (or some) of the thinking errors ask,

> *"What are the most common thinking errors or 'hot thoughts' that occur for you in challenging parenting situations? These can be thoughts about yourself, your child, or your parenting."*

Practice Challenging Thinking Errors to Feel Better

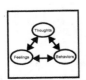

After automatic thoughts and thinking errors are identified, the next important step is to dispute the thinking errors and generate alternative thoughts for the situation (this is the "D" in Ellis' ABCD model). This is a skill that needs to be practiced! Explain to parents the process of switching from a thinking error to a more balanced thought:

> *After catching a thinking error, it is helpful to ask yourself challenge questions that will help you to come up with a different (more balanced, more helpful) thought for the situation. When you identify a different thought, you have the opportunity to feel better* [refer to CBT model if helpful]. *We will go through the thinking errors and some helpful challenge questions.*

You can refer to the second column in the table on Handout 4.1 Thinking Errors and Strategies for Increasing Helpful and Decreasing Unhelpful Thoughts to show the parent that each thinking error has challenge questions that can be used to assist in generating more helpful thoughts (i.e., positive self-talk across situations). As you discuss the following challenge questions, focus on the strategies that match up with the thinking errors discussed earlier.

Parents can challenge thinking errors by asking themselves questions like,

- *Shoulds: Can you accept yourself and others as you or they are right now? You can wish/prefer something to be the case but not demand it. Be kind to yourself and your child if you or they are not currently performing up to your standards or adjust your standards to be more realistic. (Same goes for others!)*

- *All-or-None Thinking: Does this really happen for you or your child always or never? Is this really awful? Try to think in shades of gray. Are there examples of times when this did not happen?*

- *Filtering: What are the positive parts about your parenting or your child's behavior today? What are some of your partner's positive qualities? What went OK for your family today? Are you 100% sure that there was nothing positive that happened? (Nothing is too small to count!)*

- *Labeling: Do you, your co-parent, or someone else really fit the definition of this label (e.g., lazy, loser, selfish, failure)? Are there examples that do not fit that label? Think of things as more temporary (this time, sometimes) and changeable rather than a hard and fast label.*

- *Disqualifying the Positive: What good things happened for you or your child today that you are forgetting? Are you focusing too much on one detail?*

- *Jumping to Conclusions: Is your prediction reasonable? How often are you right when you jump to the conclusion that something bad will happen?*

- *Catastrophizing: How likely is the "worst-case" scenario? What is more likely to happen? If something bad does happen, how would you handle it?*

- *Mind Reading: How do you know for sure what others are thinking? What are some more likely interpretations of the situation? What would you tell a friend who has this thought?*

- *Emotional Reasoning: What are the facts in this situation? Is this feeling leading to a helpful action? What would you tell a friend who is feeling this way?*

- *Personalization: What are you actually responsible for in this situation? What factors are out of your control? What is a fair assessment of your part?"*

You can now give the parent Worksheet 4.2: Practice Hot Thoughts and Thinking Errors, to complete as an in-session practice (Ellis & Grieger, 1986).

Group Option 1: Ask for a volunteer to go through a recent example in which they state the situation (what happened?), automatic thoughts that led to strong feelings, what thinking errors they had, and replacement thoughts (use the preceding questions to help identify replacement thoughts). For parents who are flooded with negative automatic thoughts that they take as real and valid, it is sometimes useful to engage other group members in disputing these thoughts and providing alternative, more helpful thoughts.

Group Option 2: You can go back to the list of common thoughts that the parents reported in relation to their parenting and their children on the board and have the group label the thinking errors and identify relevant challenge questions.

Therapist Note: Back to Ellis' ABCD Method

As you are discussing these challenge questions and helping parents come up with more adaptive thoughts, it is important to point out that statements about parent wishes, preferences, and likes or dislikes are perfectly reasonable. With these thoughts, parents may be annoyed or disappointed when the situation occurs, but they are unlikely to feel prolonged anger, hurt, or sadness. When challenging hot thoughts, you can incorporate the ABCD approach and try to get to the core beliefs about themselves ("I am . . . "), the world ("In a world that is . . . "), and others ("Where people are . . . ") (Persons, 1989). Rather than asking parents to immediately dispute negative thoughts, engage the person in exploring these thoughts at a deeper level using standard Beck techniques (e.g., what does it mean if . . . , what would be so bad about . . .). This approach helps get to core dysfunctional beliefs. See Beck (2011) for additional reading about these techniques.

Parents as Models: Helping Children with Thinking Errors

You can also help parents to understand that, just as adults have these automatic thinking errors, so do children. When their child says "We

NEVER get to do what I want!" that's all-or-none thinking. Children have big emotional reactions when they experience thinking errors.

It is very hard for children to change their thinking when experiencing intense emotions. Children learn about emotion regulation by watching their parents manage emotions. Parents can be models by saying out loud what their automatic thought is and then saying a more helpful thought to replace it. They can use opportunities (which are developmentally appropriate) to demonstrate changing from *first thought* to *second thought*.

For example, if a parent is disappointed because plans don't work out, they can say out loud, "I feel so disappointed. My first thought was that our day is *ruined* because we can't go on a bike ride like we planned. But then I asked myself, 'is it really that bad that my whole day is ruined?' No! My second thought is that we can find something fun to do inside and go on a bike ride tomorrow." Or "I feel frustrated! My first thought was that we *never* get a parking spot right away. But then I asked myself, 'do I really never get a parking spot right away?' No! My second thought is that we'll find a parking spot soon, and I can enjoy the music in the car until we find one." Or "My second thought is *sometimes* I get a spot right away and *sometimes* I have to wait." (See Module 9 for additional information about emotion coaching.)

When children demonstrate flexible thinking, it is an opportunity to praise them and reinforce the fact that *when we are flexible we feel better.* Noticing successes with flexibility (when a child is not upset) helps to build this skill for children, and it is easier to learn about flexibility when children are calm. When children are very upset, adults often want to challenge unhelpful thinking right away ("Of course that's not true!" or "This isn't a big deal!"). When children feel very upset, it is the *hardest* time for them to learn and practice a skill. Instead, encourage parents to help their child build the skill of flexible and helpful thinking by (1) being a model, (2) catching successes, and (3) talking about thinking errors and helpful thinking after their child has calmed down. If parents focus on being a model—catching their own thinking errors and changing to more flexible thinking—they will be in a better position to help their child.

Parents should become aware of when they may inadvertently model patterns of negative thinking for their children. Learning to counter their negative thoughts, modeling praise, and focusing on the positives can teach the child to do the same. Parents will learn more about helping their child with emotions in Module 9.

Goal 4: Teach ways to increase helpful thinking and reduce unhelpful thinking

After parents become more aware of negative patterns of thinking and specific thinking errors, they can benefit from specific strategies to help them increase flexible and helpful thinking and decrease thinking errors. More information about the strategies listed here can be found in "Control Your Depression" by Peter Lewinsohn.

Four strategies to *decrease unhelpful thoughts* are:

1. thought interruption,
2. rubber band technique,
3. worry time, and
4. the blow-up technique.

Four strategies to *increase helpful thoughts* are:

1. writing down positive self-talk statements (priming),
2. using cues,
3. writing down successes at the end of each day, and
4. time projection.

Practicing a variety of strategies will help parents to determine what works best for them, and often they will find that it is a combination of strategies that is most effective in changing thinking patterns.

Strategies to Decrease Unhelpful Thoughts

Strategy One: Thought Interruption

You can teach parents how to gain more control over their thinking by interrupting the patterns of thinking that are most common for them.

*One strategy that can help change patterns of thinking is **thought interruption**. When you notice a thinking error or unhelpful thought, INTERRUPT it with another thought. For example, if you notice you are saying to yourself "Nothing ever works out" after a challenging* *situation, is this helpful? If it isn't, yell: STOP! You can do this out loud if you are alone or in your mind if you're not. Even in your mind, try to yell loudly. Instead of STOP! you can also say to yourself, "I'm not going to think that right now" out loud or silently to yourself.*

Strategy Two: Rubber Band Technique

To have a physical reminder, some people find it helpful to wear a rubber band on their wrist and snap it when they notice a negative thought, to help interrupt it. It's a good idea to have rubber bands available if a parent wants to practice for the remainder of the session.

Strategy Three: Worry Time

Many times, our unhelpful thoughts are worries. Worries about things that are out of our control or imagining "worst-case" outcomes before anything has even happened are unhelpful and lead us to feel anxious and irritable. For example, worrying repeatedly about how a child will behave years from now is not helpful. Worries can be helpful if they lead to an action that keeps someone safe (i.e., worrying about a child running into the street leads to keeping a close eye on the child) or if they help someone to prepare (i.e., worrying about how a meeting will go leads to preparing for it). If worrying does not lead to a helpful action, it is likely a useless or unhelpful worry.

> *Worry is helpful when it leads to a helpful action. For example, worrying about your child's friendships can lead to planning a playdate in a way that your child will be most successful (time-limited, structured, etc.). However, many worries are unhelpful because we focus on things out of our control or we catastrophize (you can refer back to this thinking error). To help decrease these unhelpful worries, you can schedule a time to worry—**worry time**—and limit your worrying to this time. If a worry thought that is not helpful comes up outside of worry time, remind yourself that it is not worry time and move on. You can write the thought in a notebook or in the notes on your mobile phone if you are afraid you won't remember the worry. Your worry time should be 30 minutes at most. It's important to ONLY worry during your worry time. If you find yourself distracted and thinking about other things during worry time, make*

yourself go back to worrying. And when it's not worry time, make sure you stop yourself from worrying unless it is leading to an immediate, helpful action.

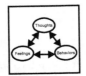

Strategy Four: Blow-up Technique

When we are stressed or anxious, we often imagine negative outcomes that are not likely to happen. To train your brain to recognize this pattern of unhelpful thinking, you can take your thoughts to a ridiculous extreme to gain more control of your thinking. Taking the negative thought to the most ridiculous extreme can often reduce the power of the thought (and even make you laugh) which can change how you feel (you can refer back to CBT model).

[You can give an example like going from the thought "our house is never clean" to imagining your house being extremely filthy and someone very important stops by unexpectedly and everything that could go wrong does.]

Strategies to Increase Helpful Thoughts

Now we will discuss four ways to increase helpful thoughts.

Strategy One: Write Down Positive Self-Talk (Priming)

Parents' thoughts can also be influenced by practicing positive self-talk several times throughout the day. Examples of self-talk include "I am doing the best I can," "I am a good mother," "My partner helps as much as they can." By writing down thoughts that are positive, helpful, and grateful, parents can increase their positive self-talk and feel better. Practicing positive self-talk on a regular basis "primes" thinking and is important in helping the thoughts to become more "automatic."

Strategy Two: Use Cues

You can remember to read the thoughts throughout the day by cueing, or pairing this with other activities, like brushing your teeth or eating (we also refer to this as "habit stacking"). You can put sticky notes on mirrors and on the refrigerator to remind you or set the timer on your phone to go off several times a day. This will help you to remember.

To practice strategies one and two to increase positive thoughts, hand out index cards and have the parent write one positive thought (or positive self-talk) on each card. They can also write thoughts on sticky notes or in the notepad of their phone. Parents can set the alarm on their phone for multiple times per day to prompt them. Encourage parents to write down thoughts about themselves, their family, and their parenting.

Group Option: Have parents share helpful thoughts and cues they have chosen to use.

Strategy Three: Pay Attention to Your Successes

When parents feel stressed, down, or anxious, positive aspects of the day can be filtered out (thinking error) and successes can be dismissed or not counted. When expectations for themselves, their child, or their parenting are unreasonable, they need to practice giving themselves credit for what *is* happening that is positive or a sign of progress.

At the end of every day, write down three things that went well that day. This can be something on your "to-do" list, something you handled well, progress you made on a goal, and so on. The important thing to remember is that nothing is too small! Some people also find it very helpful to keep a gratitude journal and to write down three things they are grateful for every day. For a related exercise, you can also do the "Favorite part of the day" ritual with your children. You can ask children what their favorite part of the day was, and then you can share what your favorite part of the day was. These practices help "train your brain" to not filter out the good parts and to notice how you feel when you change your thinking.

Strategy Four: Time Projection

When we are upset, we often think of things as being permanent rather than temporary. We can remind ourselves that things change (the only constant in life is change!), and imagining a future without a current stressor can help us to feel better now.

> *When you are in the midst of dealing with a really difficult situation, sometimes it's useful to think forward to an easier time when the stressor will no longer be there. In using time projection, you try to imagine a time when your current problem will be gone. For example, if you have a deadline at work, it sometimes helps to be able to envision yourself a little down the road, in a better place than where you are right now.*

Thoughts About the Likelihood that Parenting or Child Behavior Will Change in Treatment

Changing thoughts is hard, and you want to acknowledge that parents may be having doubts about their ability to feel better or to successfully use the strategies taught in this program.

> *The skills we talked about today take a lot of practice, so do your best to stick with them. As you practice the strategies, you might have thoughts like, "This isn't working" or you may predict, "This won't work for me." Use this as an opportunity to identify thinking errors (fortune telling, all-or-nothing thinking) and identify helpful thoughts. Examples of helpful thoughts are, "These skills have worked for others and may work for me" or "I will practice the skills regularly and see what happens." The thought "I can change my thoughts to change how I feel" can be a helpful and important thought to help you remember the reason for using the skills.*

You can also introduce the use of **mindfulness** (refer to Module 5) as parents learn more about challenging and changing thoughts. Mindfulness is being aware of what's happening in the present moment (with acceptance). This allows for a pause between our *initial reactions* (intense feelings, extreme thoughts, physiological symptoms of stress) and *our response*. This program gives parents strategies to strengthen their relationship with their child and increase appropriate behavior. However, the use of these strategies requires the parent to *respond* in the presence of strong reactions. Parents may experience muscle tension and negative thoughts about their child or parenting ("He doesn't care if he bothers others" or "Nothing works") that can prevent them from using praise to help their child. If parents practice mindfulness and improve their ability to notice their experience (and their child's experience) with acceptance, they will be more likely to respond to their child with praise despite strong reactions. If parents already have a mindfulness practice, encourage them to use this as they work to increase praises. If they have not practiced mindfulness before, there is some mindfulness instruction included in Module 5.

Throughout this program you will acknowledge the parents' own experience in challenging situations with their child so they can attend to their own needs. It is important to do this in a compassionate and validating way.

Home Practice

At the end of each session, distribute the Parent Module Summary and reinforce the fact that the information discussed today will now be practiced at home. Home practice for this module includes:

- Completing Worksheet 4.3: Looking at Connections: My Mood/Stress, Caregiving, Activities, and Thoughts
- Completing Worksheet 4.4: Special Time and Child Behavior Record Form

Discuss with parents that there is a new column on the monitoring form (Worksheet 4.3) so they can begin to track their practice of the thought strategies discussed today. Ask parents which strategies they plan to practice to increase helpful thoughts and decrease unhelpful thoughts and what will support their practice this week.

Also talk with parents about incorporating the specific (labeled) praises during Special Time practice this week. Help parents think of "positive opposites" to praise during this time. There is also an additional column on the Special Time and Child Behavior record form (Worksheet 4.4) for parents to write down their thoughts during Special Time.

This is a lot of home practice to discuss! Some parents may have difficulty keeping up with the home practice assignments. Taking time to help parents set home practice goals is important. For example, if a parent was only able to practice Special Time twice a week for the past 2 weeks, help them set a realistic goal for the next week (e.g., 3 or 4 times) and problem-solve around how to make that happen. Setting a daily phone alarm as a reminder, tying practice to a certain time of day (e.g., right after dinner), or discussing how to have a co-parent or someone else support the parent if possible (e.g., the co-parent can spend time with the sibling while the parent does Special Time) are all possible strategies to discuss.

CHAPTER 5	Module 5: Planned Ignoring and Relaxation Skills

(Recommended Length: 1 or 2 Sessions)

Materials Needed for the Module

Forms, parent summaries, worksheets, and handouts appear in Appendix A: Client Materials, located at the end of this therapist guide. You may photocopy this material for your clients, or you may download these items from the Treatments ThatWork web site at www.oxfordclinicalpsych.com/ ADHDparenting. For an outline of this and all modules, go to Appendix B: Therapist Outlines.

Parent Materials

- Module 5 Parent Summary
- Worksheet 5.1: Special Time and Child Behavior Record Form
- Worksheet 5.2: Looking at Connections: My Mood/Stress, Caregiving, Activities, and Thoughts
- The Benson Procedure script available at http://www.relaxationresponse. org/steps/
- Handout 5.1: Progressive Muscle Relaxation (PMR)
- Handout 5.2: Mindfulness

■ Form B: Top Problems

Home Practice Review from Module 4

In Module 4, parents learned to give positive attention and specific praise for effort and progress to increase appropriate and desirable behaviors. They also learned that their own automatic thoughts about their child, parenting, and self can influence how they feel and behave. Review the worksheets the parent completed tracking their pleasant activities, daily mood ratings, and Special Time. If parents did not practice at home, spend time reviewing the rationale for the home practice and help them to trouble shoot any problems they encountered. You can use some of the following questions to facilitate the home practice review.

Positive Attending

■ *How did you do with attending to your child's positive behavior? Was it easier or harder than you expected? Did you have any difficulty we can troubleshoot here?*

■ *How did it feel to be more positive with your child?*

■ *Did you notice any new thoughts about your child as a result of attending to their positive behavior?*

■ *Did you notice a positive spiral in which your behavior, thoughts, and feelings all moved in a more positive direction? How did your child react?*

■ *Did you notice any effect on your child's behavior or your relationship?*

Parents may or may not see an immediate effect on child behavior. They should be told not to be discouraged as the method may take longer to yield benefits for some children, especially if the parent–child relationship has been negative for some time. The true impact will be judged in the weeks to come as a result of its effects on the parents' own attending skills and on the parent–child relationship.

Automatic Thoughts and Changing Thoughts Strategies

- *Did you notice any examples of positive or negative spirals this week? What did you learn from the thought monitoring exercise?*
- *What are your common positive thoughts about yourself, your parenting, or your child? How about negative thoughts?*
- *Are there certain thoughts that have a more powerful effect on how you feel or behave?*
- *Are there certain times or places, or are you with certain people, when you have these thoughts, either positive or negative? (Antecedents)*
- *What helped you to manage or control your positive and negative thoughts?*

Therapist Note

Make sure to adjust the home practice review based on what was assigned in the previous session. If topics haven't been covered yet, omit the questions about that content from the home practice review. Also, if this home practice review does not include content that has been covered and assigned for home practice (e.g., if you are doing modules in a different order), make sure to expand the home practice review to include all assigned items.

Overall Module 5 Goals and Rationale

During Module 5, parents learn to use differential attention for handling minor misbehavior. They will learn the benefits of active ignoring to reduce negative attention and to improve interactions with their child by focusing attention relatively more on positive versus negative child behavior. Relative to children without attention-deficit/hyperactivity disorder (ADHD), children with ADHD and emotion regulation difficulties demonstrate a higher frequency of behaviors that parents may find annoying or disruptive, including behaviors such as tantrums, arguing, and yelling. If parents respond to *all* of these annoying behaviors, parent–child interactions will become disproportionately negative. For this reason, in this session we encourage parents to choose their battles. It will help parents to develop a *proactive* (rather than reactive) plan for those behaviors they will actively ignore and a clear understanding of why ignoring is the most effective strategy for those behaviors. The parents' use of active ignoring will be more influential now that they are regularly giving positive attention during Special Time and using labeled praise more frequently throughout the day to increase cooperative and prosocial behaviors.

That said, it is very difficult to ignore attention-seeking and emotional behaviors—the function of these behaviors is often to *get* people to pay attention or to draw attention from others. Some parents may be particularly reactive and have difficulty managing their own emotions when their child is behaving in a way the parent finds annoying or otherwise upsetting. Thus, in Module 5, parents also learn relaxation and mindfulness skills to help them be less reactive to child misbehaviors and more successful with active ignoring. The parents' own improved emotion regulation after using relaxation skills will also help them connect with and provide positive attention to their child as soon as possible following the use of active ignoring.

Specific goals for this module include

- **Goal 1:** Review with parents how much their child is motivated to earn their attention and how their attention can influence behavior.
- **Goal 2:** Help parents to choose their battles by using active ignoring for mildly annoying behaviors, attention-seeking behaviors, and emotional behaviors while maintaining high rates of praise for positive behaviors.
- **Goal 3:** Help parents to successfully implement differential attention to reduce attention-seeking behaviors and increase appropriate behavior.
- **Goal 4:** Explain the benefits of using relaxation strategies for parents to stay calm and follow through consistently with the planned ignoring skill.
- **Goal 5:** Practice strategies to help parents experience the benefits of calm breathing, PMR, and mindfulness meditation.

> *Goal 1: Review with parents how much their child is motivated to earn their attention and how their attention can influence behavior*

Begin this module by reviewing the ABC model and reminding parents that their attention is almost always a positive consequence that will encourage a child behavior (even if that behavior is negative). Parents should be very familiar with this concept from earlier modules. You can say something like,

> *We have talked about how motivating your attention is for your child. [Draw the ABC model and write "Attention" under "Consequences" with a plus sign indicating that it increases a behavior.] Whether or not we mean to do this, sometimes children get more attention from adults (parents, teachers) when they misbehave versus when they are behaving appropriately. Attention is almost always rewarding for a child—even if the quality of that attention is negative, like parents yelling, criticizing, or arguing. So giving attention to a particular child behavior actually increases the chances that the child will behave that way again in the future. For some kids, over time, they get more attention with misbehavior than for appropriate behavior.*

> *Something we refer to as "differential attention" (also called "active ignoring") can help to correct this imbalance and allow your child to receive more attention for appropriate behavior (as opposed to receiving attention for inappropriate behavior). What you pay attention to "grows," so by attending more to the positives and less to the negatives, you will encourage your child to behave appropriately in the future. Differential attention will also help your relationship with your child because it will reduce your negative feedback and therefore your negative interactions in the long run.*

Therapist Note

If parents indicate that their child's behavior does not seem to be influenced by praise, you can agree that praise alone may not be enough to address the behavioral concern. In fact, research has

---

shown that children with ADHD rarely respond to a system consisting of praise or positive consequences alone and most often need to incorporate negative consequences (like time out or privilege removal). Reassure parents that other reinforcement and consequence methods will also be taught in future sessions (e.g., Modules 7 and 10). For now, encourage parents to use their praise and attention where possible to encourage appropriate behaviors, improve child self-esteem, and improve the parent–child relationship.

Goal 2: Help parents to choose their battles by using active ignoring for mildly annoying behaviors, attention-seeking behaviors, and emotional behaviors while maintaining high rates of praise for positive behaviors

Next, introduce the concept of "planned ignoring" as a consequence that can decrease some negative behaviors in the long run (in line with the ABC Model). Early in the discussion, you can emphasize that certain behaviors should never be ignored, including noncompliance, aggression, disrespect, and other more serious rule-breaking behaviors. In these situations, ignoring the behavior can result in someone being hurt. Teach parents that active ignoring is an effective consequence for mildly annoying, disruptive, or emotional behaviors that are not more serious, like rule-breaking and aggression. Many children with ADHD exhibit hyperactive and impulsive behaviors like making noises, fidgeting, talking loudly/constantly, and tapping, as well as emotional behaviors like complaining, whining, or begging when feeling upset. These more minor behaviors may annoy parents, especially when they are feeling stressed or irritable. These are the types of minor misbehaviors that are very appropriate to ignore.

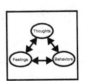

By ignoring some of these mild and annoying behaviors, parents can accomplish a lot of good things. First, interactions should feel less negative when parents reduce criticism and correction for every little thing. Instead, they'll be choosing their battles and only responding with negative attention to the more serious negative behaviors. Second, their child will learn that positive behavior, rather than negative behavior, will receive parental attention. Finally, the parent may *feel* and *think* more positively about their child as they give less attention to mild negative behaviors (tie in with Module 4). Tipping the balance of parent–child interactions in favor of the positives (as opposed to the negatives) should leave both the parent and child feeling better. You can say something like,

Just as attention increases the chances that a behavior will occur again, active ignoring or intentionally removing your attention from minor misbehaviors can decrease the likelihood that a behavior will continue. [Add "Active Ignoring or Remove Attention" under "Consequences" in the ABC model previously drawn. Put a minus sign indicating that it decreases behavior.] *This is especially true for mild inappropriate behaviors such as making noises during meals or homework, squirming or fidgeting rather than sitting still, interrupting you when you are in a conversation, or continuing to argue or negotiate when your child has already been given an answer.*

What are situations where your child makes noise, interrupts, or does other mildly annoying or emotional behaviors that may get your attention?

Make sure that the parent is choosing behaviors that are appropriate for ignoring. If they suggest a behavior that is rule-breaking or aggressive and should not be ignored, let them know that ignoring more serious behaviors can mean that their child is avoiding a consequence, which makes it more likely for that behavior to happen again. Someone (e.g., a sibling) can also get hurt!

If there is more than one parent or caregiver in the home, they need to come to an agreement on which behaviors will be ignored. Consistency across time and caregivers is one of the most important elements related to the success of planned ignoring and this program more generally.

For some situations, it is easier for children to get attention for disruptive behavior rather than appropriate behaviors like waiting, playing independently, or being flexible/accepting when the answer is no. To illustrate this, give the example of a child's interrupting behaviors getting attention during a parent phone call rather than the parent temporarily stopping the call to give attention for patience and waiting. Normalize that less attention is often given to children when they are playing or complying and *not* disrupting. Children are often most successful at obtaining parental attention or getting what they want when they disrupt parent activities, particularly if that activity involves attention being paid to someone else other than the child. This is a common cycle and one that parents can change when they are proactive and catch behaviors related to self-regulation and cooperation before a problem behavior begins.

> *Goal 3: Help parents to successfully implement differential attention to reduce attention seeking behaviors and increase appropriate behavior*

For active ignoring to be effective, the concept of *differential attention* can now be explained. Both positive attention and ignoring need be done *in combination* so that the child can effectively learn which behaviors receive parent attention and which do not. Ignoring misbehavior without positive attention for desired (expected) behaviors will not be as effective, and the balance toward the negative will remain. You can help parents to think of ignoring as a "withdrawal," and they need to fill the child's "bank account" with positive attention at other times. For example, parents should take every opportunity to praise the positive opposite of problem behaviors, such as working quietly or accepting a limit with calm behavior, as we discussed in Module 4.

In addition, both strategies (praise and ignoring) must be used *consistently* to be effective. If attention-seeking behaviors are attended to even *some* of the time, they will persist. You can provide information about the power of intermittent reinforcement (similar to payouts from a slot machine) to help parents understand why behaviors continue even if they respond to them effectively most of the time.

What Exactly Is Meant by Active Ignoring?

Explain to the parent that active ignoring means no eye contact, no verbal contact, and no physical contact with their child until the behavior ends. You can ask the parent what their child's reaction may be to ignoring and emphasize the notion that it is likely for the child to up the ante and increase the intensity of their misbehavior to try to obtain the parent's attention or get what the child wants. In classic behavioral theory, this is referred to as the *extinction burst*. The parent needs to be prepared for this temporary escalation of negative behavior and commit to ignoring *until the behavior stops*. If the behavior escalates and the parent gives in at that point, the child learns that the persistence and/or escalation of misbehavior is what worked and thus the child learns to display the misbehavior at a *more intense* level in the future (e.g., whining, crying, or yelling more loudly or intensely). The classic example is a child tantruming in the grocery store when the parent says no to a request for candy at the checkout line. If the parent tries to ignore but then gives in when the behavior becomes louder (and therefore more embarrassing), the child has learned that the misbehavior (and escalation/persistence) is rewarded.

This can also be a good time to illustrate the option of marked "candy free aisles" as a great antecedent that makes it less likely that the child will demand candy in the first place. Another antecedent would be the parent reviewing the rules and expectations prior to entering the grocery store (discussed in detail in Module 7).

Another important part of differential attention is for the parent to be looking for the first opportunity to praise the child for behaving appropriately. That is, once the child has stopped the negative behavior, the parent should praise the child for the first appropriate behavior the parent notices. The contrast between the parent's response to the mildly inappropriate behavior (ignoring) versus the appropriate behavior (praising) should be loud and clear!

Throughout the program we are putting a complicated puzzle together in order to best help the family with their Top Problems. It can be helpful to highlight how the "pieces" (in this case antecedents and consequences) fit together. This also helps parents to have appropriate expectations and not expect one piece (strategy) to fix the problem.

Given the difficult history that some parents have had with trying ignoring, you can say

One thing to keep in mind is that ignoring may be one of the most difficult skills to use effectively because you may feel like you have to do something when your child behaves inappropriately and the behavior can get more intense in the short-term. The problem is that you have plenty to deal with in terms of inappropriate or problematic behavior!

You can afford to choose your battles and ignore minor, attention-seeking behaviors. And, in many cases, removing your attention until the behavior ends is the most effective way to influence that behavior. You are using your attention strategically.

Emphasize to the parent that the key to this skill is *consistency*: consistency between caregivers, ignoring each and every time the behavior occurs, and following through until the very end of the episode (e.g., tantrum). Help parents select at least two specific behaviors on which they plan to use the active ignoring strategy for this week. Help them anticipate potential challenges that may arise and how they may address this. It can be helpful to role-play active ignoring in session, particularly with parents who may have difficulty being assertive or who may have a harder time refraining from giving negative attention.

Parents may have concerns about others' reactions to their use of active ignoring, which can be perceived by others as not addressing a behavior. Help parents to problem-solve how they will handle the reactions of others in situations where active ignoring will be helpful for their child. Make sure to identify any concerns that may contribute to inconsistency between caregivers. You can also let parents know that you will be teaching assertiveness skills in Module 6 because a common concern is how to communicate effectively with others in challenging parenting situations.

Group Option: Have the group generate ideas for positive opposites of the child behaviors that group members chose for ignoring this week. Group members can also pair up to practice planned ignoring by role-playing a common situation they encounter with their children (e.g., tantrum, complaining).

Goal 4: Explain the benefits of using relaxation strategies for parents to stay calm and follow through consistently with the planned ignoring skill

Next, introduce three techniques for parents to use to help with their own emotion regulation and relaxation in tough parenting situations. Knowing *how to relax* can help parents to remain calm and neutral in discipline situations with their child. In this module, we will focus on helping parents to see the value of improving their ability to relax in order to successfully ignore misbehavior that can be very irritating or frustrating for them. The skill of relaxation will also be useful in several future modules, such as Modules 7 (Time Out) and 8 (Working with the Schools), as well as in managing stressors outside of parenting. In addition, tension can contribute to parents' mood, anxiety, or stress more generally by making it difficult for them to enjoy activities in their lives. By learning and practicing ways to feel calm and relaxed, parents can influence their feelings and thoughts. Parents can also benefit from practicing mindfulness so they can bring this present moment awareness and acceptance into parenting and self-care activities.

There are now "mindful parenting" programs (Bögels & Restifo, 2014) to help parents bring nonjudgmental attention to their parenting, children, and themselves.

Spend a little time within the session asking parents about their past experience and/or current use of relaxation, deep breathing, and mindfulness/meditation. If helpful, assist the parent in identifying any *thoughts* that may influence their motivation or ability to see the possible benefits of relaxation or to practice this skill.

> ### Goal 5: Practice strategies to help parents experience the benefits of calm breathing, PMR, and mindfulness meditation

Teach three different relaxation techniques that can help in tense parenting situations, such as when parents need to follow through or ignore an irritating behavior: (1) a passive, portable, *meditative breathing* method developed by Benson (Benson, Beary, & Carol, 1974; Lewinsohn, Munoz, Youngren, & Zeiss, 1986), (2) *Jacobson's Progressive Muscle Relaxation* (PMR; Jacobson, 1929), and (3) *mindfulness meditation*, which can be defined as "paying attention in a particular way; on purpose, in the present moment and nonjudgmentally" (Kabat-Zinn, 1994). By presenting three options, the idea is for parents to try all of them and ultimately choose the one that is the best fit and/or most helpful for them. Some parents may have prior experience with one of the three approaches, in which case they may just want to resume their practice. They may also decide to use more than one approach at different times.

Let parents know that all of these methods are highly effective and to expect that the methods will become more beneficial the more the parents practice. You can also share that there are a variety of apps that can help with relaxation practice (such as Insight Timer, Calm, and Headspace for guided meditations). If relevant to the parents, smartphones and smartwatches also have features to remind us to practice calm breathing throughout the day. Establishing the habit of relaxation practice is like building a parachute—by practicing regularly, the parents will have this skill available during their most challenging moments (when the parachute is needed!). Another analogy is the need for scuba divers to practice skills repeatedly on dry land before they practice in a challenging situation in the water. Parents should try to practice some form of relaxation at least once or twice a day *when they are calm*. As they gain experience with these relaxation strategies, they can more effectively use them when they are stressed (e.g., when trying to ignore the child's annoying behaviors).

The first of these approaches is the **Benson Procedure.** This approach involves focusing on the breath moving in and out while repeating a meditative word (such as "one," "peace," or "om"). Relaxation methods focused on the breath are helpful because they can be done almost anywhere and at any time. Let the parent know that at first it is helpful to practice in a calm environment without distractions. After parents practice and the technique becomes more automatic and easier, they will be able to use it in more challenging situations with their children and in other areas of their life. You can use the Benson Procedure script available at http://www.relaxationresponse.org/steps/ to guide the practice. Practice for at least 5 minutes in session to make sure you can address any questions or concerns.

Encourage parents to use a passive attitude while practicing relaxation breathing. Instruct them to not judge whether they are doing it right or whether they are able to relax. Also normalize the experience of distracting thoughts that come during relaxation practice. These distracting thoughts occur for almost everyone, especially as they are beginning their practice. When experience a distracting thought, suggest to the parent that they go back to their word/breath. They can also envision the thought floating away like a leaf down a creek or like a cloud across the sky. Keeping a "let it happen" attitude is one of the most important elements in becoming deeply relaxed. Remember, staying focused during relaxation practice is a skill that develops over time. Encourage parents to stick with it in order to derive full benefit. As noted, there are apps on smartphones and watches to guide breathing practice, many of which include alerts or reminders to prompt daily practice.

The second relaxation technique you will teach parents is Jacobson's **PMR**, which involves tensing and relaxing different muscle groups in succession. PMR is useful because it helps us to notice the difference between the feelings of relaxation and feelings of tension in our bodies. You can use Handout 5.1: Progressive Muscle Relaxation (PMR) to guide the practice. Before the PMR practice (which should happen in session), ask the parent to give you a rating of tension from 1–10, with 10 being the most tense (e.g., lion is chasing you) and 1 being the most relaxed (e.g., lying on a beach). After the practice, ask parents to again give their tension rating. You can have them share about areas of their body where they noticed tension and any challenges they experienced during the practice (like distracting thoughts, sleepiness, or discomfort). During the week, they can tune in to these areas from time to time to gauge how tense or relaxed they are throughout the day. Tension in one of these areas can prompt them to practice their relaxation techniques.

Parents may wish to use a PMR app to guide their practice. There are also many good PMR videos available on YouTube.

The third technique to teach parents is **mindfulness meditation** (see Handout 5.2: Mindfulness). By practicing mindfulness meditation, parents can learn to notice their present moment experience without judgment. There are different ways to practice mindfulness, but they share a focus on noticing what is happening (thoughts, feelings, sensations) with acceptance. Practice can include:

1. *Notice your senses.* A common mindfulness practice is to notice 5 things you see, 4 things you can touch, 3 things you hear, 2 things you can smell, and 1 thing you can hear. You can also focus on one sense: look for things that are blue or a certain shape; only attend to one sense like sound and keep bringing awareness back to sound.
2. *Do an activity mindfully.* Common daily activities like walking, eating, drinking, showering, brushing your teeth, even washing dishes can be done with mindful awareness of the experience. During

the activity you notice sensations and give your full attention to the experience. When you eat or drink mindfully, you notice the taste, texture, and temperature as you eat. If you become distracted by thoughts, you gently bring your attention back to the experience. When you brush your teeth mindfully you are aware of the taste and sensations of brushing with no judgment. If you wash dishes you notice the sights, sounds, and sensations of touching the water, soap, and dishes.

3. *Mindfulness meditation*. Focus on your breath going in and out. When you notice thinking, let thoughts go rather than follow the thought (or ruminate), push the thought away, or focus on the thought (which can intensify feelings). To let thoughts go, imagine the thought floating away like a leaf down the creek or like a cloud across the sky.

Home Practice

At the end of each session, distribute the Parent Module Summary and reinforce the fact that the information discussed today will now be practiced at home. Home practice for this module includes:

- Completing Worksheet 5.1: Special Time and Child Behavior Record Form
- Completing Worksheet 5.2: Looking at Connections: My Mood/ Stress, Caregiving, Activities, and Thoughts

Differential Attention

Before ending the session, the parent should have identified two minor, irritating child behaviors they are going to work to ignore this week. The first thing the parent should do is to discuss with their co-parent (if relevant) whether they also feel comfortable ignoring this behavior. This has to be a joint decision because consistency is key!

Remind the parent to keep praising the child for their positive behaviors. For instance, the parent should take time to praise the child when the child is working or playing independently rather than waiting until the child misbehaves.

Finally, remind parents that the behavior they are trying to ignore may escalate, or increase in severity, when they are ignoring. They should continue to ignore until the behavior decreases; otherwise, they will be teaching the child to start out at a higher intensity of misbehavior in the future.

Relaxation

Encourage parents to practice their relaxation skills once per day (for about 10–15 minutes) to begin, recognizing that it will become easier with practice. They may start out trying a variety of the skills reviewed in this module or focus on the approach they feel is the best fit for them. They should begin by practicing during a quiet time of day, such as bedtime or when they first wake up. They can schedule this practice on their calendar and set alerts/reminders to enhance follow through (see Module 3). Eventually, as they get better at it, parents can use these relaxation skills to help them stay cool when using planned ignoring. Remind parents to continue to monitor their mood and activities. They may notice that they are able to enjoy activities more when they are feeling more relaxed.

Finally, remind parents again that relaxation is a skill that develops with regular practice. Like any other skill, it takes time to develop, so they should not be discouraged if it takes awhile to feel comfortable with the procedures, being able to focus, and so on.

CHAPTER 6

Module 6: Assertiveness, Effective Commands, and House Rules

(Recommended Length: 2 Sessions; one for Assertiveness and one for Commands and House Rules)

Materials Needed for the Module

Forms, parent summaries, worksheets, and handouts appear in Appendix A: Client Materials, located at the end of this therapist guide. You may photocopy this material for your clients, or you may download these items from the Treatments ThatWork web site at www.oxfordclinicalpsych.com/ ADHDparenting. For an outline of this and all modules, go to Appendix B: Therapist Outlines.

Parent Materials

- Module 6 Parent Summary
- Worksheet 6.1: Communication Styles
- Worksheet 6.2: Effective Commands
- Worksheet 6.3: Looking at Connections: My Mood/Stress, Caregiving, Activities, and Thoughts
- Worksheet 6.4: Special Time and Child Behavior Record Form
- Handout 6.1: Assertiveness

- Form B: Top Problems

Home Practice Review from Module 5

During Module 5, parents learned to ignore and use differential attention to handle minor misbehavior. Parents also learned relaxation skills to help them be less reactive to child misbehaviors and more successful with active ignoring and the other skills taught in this program.

Review the worksheets the parent completed tracking their Special Time, pleasant activities, daily mood ratings, thought strategies, and relaxation strategies. If parents did not practice at home, spend time reviewing the rationale for the home practice and help them to troubleshoot any problems they encountered. You can use some of the following questions to facilitate the home practice review:

- *How did the planned ignoring practice go for the behaviors you identified in our last meeting? Were you able to ignore all the way through until your child's behavior changed? Did you follow-up with a praise for appropriate behavior at the first opportunity?*
- *How did you keep your cool during ignoring?*
- *How did your relaxation practice go? Which approach worked best for you? Were you able to use relaxation in any parenting situations this week?*

It is important to remind parents that relaxation is a skill that takes practice—it may come easily to some people, and for others it may be more difficult. Relaxation might be an especially important skill for those who find it most difficult, and, like other skills, it can improve with practice. And there are many ways to relax. Parents can keep in mind that the goal is not to entirely remove all anxiety since some level of tension is known to be adaptive and necessary to function effectively. The goal is to use these strategies to develop a generally calm approach to the child, particularly when using skills like planned ignoring or time out (covered in Module 7).

> **Therapist Note**
>
> Make sure to adjust the home practice review based on what was assigned in the previous session. If topics haven't been covered yet, omit questions about that content from the home practice review. Also, if this home practice review does not include content that has been covered and assigned for home practice (e.g., if you are doing modules in a different order), make sure to expand the home practice review to include all assigned items.

Overall Module 6 Goals and Rationale

During Module 6, parents will learn about assertiveness and how to apply assertiveness skills to improve communication with others. For parenting, there are many benefits to an *assertive* parenting style. An assertive (or authoritative) parenting style provides both nurturance and structure. The assertive parent follows through with healthy boundaries in a calm and effective manner. Signs of a *permissive* parenting style include unclear or inconsistent expectations, worry about a child's reaction to discipline, and the parent feeling overly responsible for their child's emotions and behaviors when difficult situations arise. Signs of an *authoritarian* parenting style can include low warmth, many strict, rigid rules or the absence of clear expectations paired with harsh reactions when expectations are not met. Families can have elements of the three parenting styles (permissive, authoritarian, and assertive; Baumrind, 1966). Moving toward a more consistent assertive parenting style benefits all family members.

Parents also need to use their assertiveness skills when they communicate with their child's school, other caregivers, and extended family members. Parents need to communicate effectively with others so that their child receives needed support. For example, making a request to teachers, pursuing accommodations at school, asking questions of care providers (e.g., the pediatrician or child psychiatrist), and advocating for their child when others don't understand their child's needs requires assertiveness on the part of the parent. Often, as parents try to implement new parenting strategies, they may encounter disapproval from extended family members, requiring them to respond with assertiveness.

In addition, parents' success with self-care requires asserting their *own* needs (e.g., saying "no" to additional obligations), following through with needed changes, and challenging beliefs (thoughts) about holding others accountable or asking for help. Given the large influence of social interactions on mood, assertiveness skills can have significant benefits for a parent's overall interpersonal functioning across domains of family and work.

Specific goals for this module include

- **Goal 1:** Help parents identify difficulties they may have with assertiveness, both related to their parenting and the rest of their lives.
- **Goal 2:** Work with parents to increase their assertive behavior.
- **Goal 3:** Increase the effectiveness of parental commands to improve child compliance.
- **Goal 4:** Identify a few house rules that are expected of all members within the household.

Module 6 Content (Divided by Goals)

> *Goal 1: Help parents identify difficulties they may have with assertiveness, related to both their parenting and the rest of their lives*

Begin by providing information to the parent about what assertiveness is and why it is beneficial. *Assertiveness* means someone letting others know what they feel, need, or want without being aggressive or passive. It is the ability to express both pleasant and unpleasant thoughts and feelings openly. Assertiveness helps make our relationships closer, helps others understand us better, and most often leads to more positive outcomes. If someone is passive and ignores their own needs, stress will build over time and they can become resentful. If someone is aggressive, they can ignore the needs of others and be too harsh when giving feedback or setting a boundary.

As illustrated in Figure 6.1, communication exists across a continuum, with three key points: passive, assertive, and aggressive. Draw the continuum for parents to illustrate the types of communication. Explain

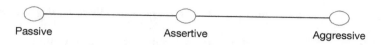

Passive　　　　　　　　　Assertive　　　　　　　　Aggressive

Figure 6.1

The communication continuum.

that we may be in different places on the continuum depending on who we are with and the demands of the situation. We can also move along the continuum based on people's reactions to us and how we are feeling at that moment. Someone may swing from passive to aggressive (and back to passive).

Point out the goal of *starting and staying assertive*. Share signs of a **passive approach** including speaking softly, slouching, minimal eye contact, blank or hesitant expression, apologizing when you have done nothing wrong, tentative language, and ignoring your own thoughts and feelings. Alternatively, signs of an **aggressive approach** can include interrupting, talking loudly, glaring, scowling, being in others' personal space, having a closed-off stance, and not considering others' feelings. Signs of **assertive communication** include speaking calmly and firmly, having a relaxed and open posture, making good eye contact, and being considerate of people's needs and feelings. In assertive communication, *boundaries* are clearly defined (you know *what is okay and not okay for yourself*), you ask for what you need (you don't wait for others to determine what you need), negative thoughts and feelings are expressed in a healthy and respectful manner, and compliments and criticisms are accepted.

You can provide some brief examples of the three communication types for the following scenarios before you have parents share more about their own communication style and when it is most difficult to communicate assertively.

Example (stressed about the amount of work to do, talking to co-parent):

- *Aggressive*: You never help out!
- *Assertive*: I am feeling overwhelmed with all of the tasks for the house and the kids. I need us to work together to share the workload.
- *Passive*: I'm sorry that I am not doing enough or I wish someone would maybe help me out (vague).

Example (child is struggling at school, talking to teacher):

- *Aggressive*: You don't care about my child.
- *Assertive*: I am concerned about how my child's challenges are affecting him in the classroom. I want to make sure he is getting the support he needs to be successful.
- *Passive*: You are the expert and know more than I do, so I will follow whatever you say.

Ask parents if they notice situations with their child, family, friends, work, or community when they have trouble being assertive. During times of stress or challenge, what passive responses do they make? What aggressive responses? You can also tie in that these communication styles are similar to the different types of parenting styles (permissive, authoritative, and authoritarian).

> **Goal 2: Work with parents to increase their assertive behavior**

Identify Situations

Next you will help parents to identify situations in which they may have difficulty with assertiveness, including interactions with their child and other situations in their lives. One situation that often comes up is that it can be difficult to say "no" to things others ask us to do (other adults or our children). This was discussed in Module 3 (time management), and it is worth revisiting in this module. Not being assertive in these situations can lead to overcommitment, which is not good for parent self-care.

Have parents Complete Worksheet 6.1: Communication Styles to help them identify their thoughts and actions associated with the three communication styles as you go through the following information.

Identify Thoughts and Actions

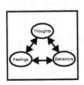
For situations when parents have more difficulty with assertive behavior, ask them to identify *thoughts* (what they are saying to themselves) that make it harder to be assertive. When we feel down, stressed, or anxious, our thinking may lead to more passive or aggressive communication.

You can then help parents to identify replacement thoughts that make assertive behavior more likely.

Examples of thoughts that can lead to passive communication, followed by a more assertive interpretation:

- Nothing ever works out → I can focus on what I can control
- Nobody cares → I can give people the chance to be helpful
- My child will hate me → My child needs healthy limits
- This person won't like me → I have the right to say no

Examples of thoughts that can lead to aggressive communication, followed by a more assertive interpretation:

- He's manipulating me → Both of our needs are valid
- She's doing this on purpose → She is having a hard time
- The school doesn't really care about my child → The school is doing its best and may not know exactly what my child needs

Ask parents what they are likely to say or do if they use assertive thoughts (mindset) in challenging situations. Compare this to what would be said or done following passive or aggressive thoughts (mindset).

Assertive Imagery

Next you will teach parents how to use assertive imagery to improve their assertiveness skills. This technique allows parents to imagine, anticipate, and practice assertive responses in their mind first, which will make it easier for them to handle these situations when they occur. The goal is to have parents gain confidence that they can handle situations that arise in the most effective way possible and that they are prepared for a range of responses from the other person/people.

To practice, have the parent create a vivid image of a situation by imagining where it occurs, who is there, and where they are in the scene. Tell the parent to imagine what each person is saying and doing and then imagine their own behavior or response. The goal is to say something assertive that satisfies them. Have them imagine what happens after they assert themselves: What would others say and do? Help them to create a vivid image of the positive effects of their assertive behavior.

The next step in the visualization practice can include the same scene with some of the details changed. For example, they can imagine a different reaction from others and how they would handle that.

Examples

Imagine someone asking you to do something and confidently and nicely saying "no." If it is hard to be assertive with your child, imagine calmly and confidently setting a limit and telling your child exactly what you will or won't do. Imagine these situations having positive outcomes. Then imagine the person responding in a difficult way and how you would handle that response assertively. Talk with parents about continuing to practice assertive imagery at home to increase their comfort and efficacy with assertiveness skills.

Next, ask parents to choose an "easy" situation (i.e., one that is most likely to be successful) to practice assertiveness in their own lives. Use Handout 6.1: Assertiveness to guide this exercise. Encourage parents to take a proactive approach and plan for the situation rather than waiting for it to happen. Remind parents that as they begin to practice assertiveness, they will need to be flexible and give themselves credit for progress (not perfection!). Convey confidence that assertiveness skills can be learned and developed, but it will take patience and practice until they feel more confident and effective in challenging social situations.

For parents who would benefit from additional instruction, you can also incorporate the *DEARMAN skill* from dialectical behavior therapy (Linehan, 1993) to help parents increase assertive communication. This skill aims to increase interpersonal effectiveness by using a specific framework for responding to requests. See Linehan (2014) for additional information.

Therapist Note

A variety of outcomes can occur when parents begin to practice assertiveness. A lack of progress can be due to a long history of being nonassertive, lack of consistent practice, and standards that are too high. The goal, again, is to help parents gain increasing comfort and confidence with asserting their feelings and needs in multiple areas of their lives.

Goal 3: Increase the effectiveness of parental commands to improve child compliance

An important area in which to apply assertiveness skills is when parents need to give their child a direction or command. By giving effective commands in an assertive way—not passively or aggressively (i.e., in a calm and neutral, yet confident, voice)—parents can take a proactive stance when they need their child to do something. Parents will now learn guidelines for effective commands that help them to be very clear and help the child to be successful. These guidelines are based on research conducted by Rex Forehand in the 1970s and 1980s that shows that the manner in which a direction is stated influences the likelihood that a child will comply (e.g., Roberts, McMahon, Forehand, & Humphreys, 1978). For children with attention and behavior problems, it is important that parents communicate clear expectations when their child needs to perform daily tasks, transition from preferred activities, and follow routines. At this time, remind parents of the ABC model of child behavior (Module 1) and show that effective commands are an antecedent that makes compliance (the behavior) more likely. To help establish parent mastery of the ABC model, also prompt parents to tell you what a helpful consequence would be for compliance (e.g., praise) to reinforce their knowledge of behavioral principles they have learned.

You will now share guidelines for effective commands that can be used as an important antecedent that can lead to improved child compliance.

The first guideline for effective commands is to make sure that the command is *necessary*. Parents should consider if the command is important enough to reinforce with praise or follow through with a consequence. If not, it is better to give the child a choice, do something for the child, or choose your battles rather than give a direction. If parents are too stressed or tired to follow through, it is better to choose a different approach (not give a command) to avoid inconsistency with following through in response to noncompliance.

Examples

- AVOID commands that aren't necessary: "Make your bed" or "Play with the blocks."

- DO commands that are necessary: "Please brush your teeth."
- DO give choices when appropriate: "Do you want to play with blocks or something else?"

The second guideline is that commands should be *stated directly* in a confident/firm but calm/neutral tone of voice. This is a good time to review the difference between passive, aggressive, and assertive approaches in the context of parenting. Asking a question (passive) implies that the child has a choice and can increase the likelihood of noncompliance. Using a harsh tone may teach the child that you don't "mean business" when commands are given with a neutral and respectful tone. A direct, clear command also tells the child what *to do* instead of what not to do. It is more clear and assertive to say, "Please put your hands by your side" rather than "Stop touching your sister."

Examples

- AVOID passive communication: "How about we clean up?"
- AVOID aggressive communication: "You better clean up right this second . . . or else!!" or "Why don't you ever do what you are told!?"
- DO use assertive communication: "Please put the toys back in the toy box" or "Please get in the shower."

Refer back to the passive-assertive-aggressive continuum of communication.

The third guideline is for parents to give *simple, one-step commands* rather than multiple steps and more complex commands. Children with inattention may struggle to remember each part of a multistep direction and may therefore only comply with some parts of a multistep direction, not because they don't want to but because they do not remember the various parts of the command. It is also hard to know how to follow-up if there is partial compliance (do you give a positive or negative consequence?). Thus, commands should be given one at a time for larger tasks or routines with multiple steps.

The command should also be mindful of the child's attentional or organizational capacity. In other words, if the child can only focus for 10–15 minutes, commands like "Clean your room" or "Clean out the garage" are problematic since these tasks could take hours. Rather, commands like "Put your dirty clothes in the hamper" or "Sweep the garage floor" would be more specific and appropriate to the child's attentional and organizational capabilities.

Examples

- AVOID large or multistep commands: "Clean up all of your toys" or "Get ready for bed."
- DO simple, one-step commands: "Please put on your pajamas" or "Please brush your teeth."

The fourth guideline is that parents should **make sure they have their child's attention** before giving a command by reducing distractions, standing close to their child, and making eye contact. It can be tempting to give commands by shouting from a different room, but ensuring that you have the child's attention before the command helps them to be successful and allows the parent to follow through immediately with praise or a negative consequence. Reducing distractions may include pausing or turning off screens, turning down the volume on music, or moving a toy. If needed, a parent can also have the child restate the command to check for understanding and to help them remember.

Examples

- AVOID distractions: "Put your shoes on" (from another room while the child is watching television).
- DO reduce distractions: "Please put your shoes on" (after turning off the television and establishing eye contact with the child).

The fifth guideline is for parents to give some time for their child to complete one direction before giving another. Thus, the **timing of a direction** can influence the child's success with compliance. Parents should wait 10 seconds to give their child a chance to listen after giving a command. During this time parents should stay quiet so they do not distract their child or nag.

Examples

- AVOID too many commands: "Put your pajamas on" (3 seconds) "And brush your teeth" (5 seconds) "And pick up your toys!"
- AVOID too much talking: "Put your pajamas on. . . . You need to get ready for bed so we have time to read books and you can get enough sleep. . . . Why aren't you getting dressed? It is getting so late!"
- DO give one command and stay quiet: "Put your pajamas on" and stay quiet for 10 seconds.

For older children who may need to complete more complicated tasks such as cleaning their bedroom or doing homework, parents and children can work together to write down the series of steps needed to successfully complete the task in checklist style, and children can check off each step when it is done. This allows the parent to reinforce the child for each successful step. For chores, a note card can be made for each chore that gives specific information about what needs to be done for the chore to be completed. This approach has the added benefit of teaching the child the process by which one breaks down tasks and makes a list for themselves. This will come in handy as they get older!

Examples

- AVOID giving one command for complicated tasks that exceed the child's attentional/organizational ability: "Do your homework" or "Clean your room."
- DO make a checklist: "The steps for cleaning your bedroom are: put clothes away, pick up toys, and empty the trash" or "Sit at homework spot at 4 PM, check planner, and get out materials for first assignment."

Give the parents Worksheet 6.2: Effective Commands to practice in session.

You will next talk with the parent about practicing at home by giving simple, direct commands that their child is very likely to do. For example, the parent can tell the child to hand them something easily within reach, put something in their backpack, or do a routine task that requires minimal effort like throwing something away in the trash or putting a dish in the sink. The parent should plan to practice commands for brief periods (a few minutes) several times a day when their child is not distracted with a preferred activity. The parent will have more opportunities to provide reinforcement for compliance if they practice giving more frequent simple commands on a daily basis this week. This will help to increase the desired behavior of compliance. You can model giving a few commands and giving attention and praise for compliance. Parents can experience a range of reactions to applying assertiveness to giving directions to their child. Often parents will anticipate or expect that their child will not comply with commands (this is a negative thought; see Module 4). Encourage them to first focus on the proactive strategy of stating directions following the guidelines reviewed today and to praise their child for compliance. In future sessions (e.g., Module 7), negative consequences will be discussed, but for now parents should continue to respond as they usually do when there is noncompliance. The focus for this week is on giving effective commands and catching and praising child compliance whenever it happens (Module 4).

Parents may also believe that praise for compliance will not be motivating for their child. You can review information from Module 4 about the influence of parental attention and praise. Encourage the parent to continue to be consistent in using labeled praise even if the impact on child behavior is not noticed immediately. Sometimes what we *don't* do is as important as what we do. If the parent is becoming more positive with their attention, they are also reducing criticism and other negative behaviors.

Last, some parents may believe that assertive commands sound too harsh or rigid. You can remind them that these guidelines aim to achieve an assertive approach to commands that sets their child up for success and ultimately helps their child with security and healthy boundaries. For children who struggle with inattention, impulsivity, low frustration tolerance, and related challenges, giving clear and direct expectations is a *form of support* and allows them to show what they are capable of doing. You can also remind parents that research shows that a more indirect or passive approach to giving commands elicits more noncompliance.

Goal 4: Identify a few house rules that are expected of all members within the household

Another aspect of assertive parenting is establishing *house rules* to let children know very specifically what is expected at all times, even before misbehavior occurs. Have parents identify house rules as an antecedent in the ABC model of child behavior (Module 1) that helps their child to demonstrate appropriate behavior. House rules are also *pro*active (rather than *re*active) because they are discussed at a neutral time when the behavior has not occurred, and the child will know exactly what to expect if and when the house rule is broken.

House rules are helpful for (1) impulsive behaviors, (2) behaviors that are never allowed, and (3) "stop" behaviors because there is not time to give a command in these situations (i.e., the behavior has already happened). House rules should make it clear to the child what behavior is not allowed. For example:

- "No hitting,"
- "No name calling,"
- "No destroying property,"
- "No touching the computer or other electronics without permission," and
- "No going outside without permission."

For this week, instruct parents to choose one to three house rules and begin to label these behaviors at home when they happen. The parent should choose behaviors that they would like for their child to demonstrate without reminders. For now, the parent should focus on establishing the rules and making sure their child understands which behaviors count as rule-breaking. In Module 7 you will teach the parent to use an immediate consequence for rule-breaking to reduce impulsive behaviors. You can let parents know that when house rules are established and the behavior is labeled for their child ("you broke a house rule"), they are beginning to help their child with self-regulation.

Talk with parents about starting the house rules at home. They can have a family meeting at a neutral time to identify the house rules together with their child(ren). They can ask children to contribute ideas for house rules, but parents have the final word. It can be helpful for parents to express that house rules are helpful for *all* family members (parents too!) such as "No mean words," "No hurting," and "No swearing."

> **Therapist Note**
>
> Some parents will want to phrase the house rules positively. Although this is admirable, we have found that positively phrased house rules are not as specific (e.g., be kind to one another), and it is critically important that the child knows exactly what is expected of them. One way to accommodate parents who are adamant about this is to allow the positively phrased rule and then add bullets underneath about what this means more specifically (e.g., no mean words, no hurting).

The house rules should be posted in a prominent place in the home. Children can help decorate the poster. Pictures are helpful for younger children who may not yet be able to read.

When parents begin to implement a new house rule, they should also increase the positive attention they give for rule following (i.e., praising the positive opposite). If the rule is "No hurting," the parent should give specific praises for being gentle, keeping their body calm when they are angry, and using words to express feelings.

Home Practice

At the end of each session, distribute the Parent Module Summary and reinforce the fact that the information discussed today will now be practiced at home. Home practice for this module includes:

- Assertiveness imagery practice and using assertive thoughts and behaviors in low demand situations where the parent can be successful
- Identify 2–3 house rules, talk to their child about the rules, and post them
- Completing Worksheet 6.3: Looking at Connections: My Mood/ Stress, Caregiving, Activities, and Thoughts
- Completing Worksheet 6.4: Special Time and Child Behavior Record Form

Show parents that there is a new column on Worksheet 6.4: Special Time and Child Behavior Record Form so they can track practicing commands this week. Parents should practice the methods for increasing the effectiveness of their commands and should implement 2–3 compliance training periods (where they give high rates of simple commands) per day. Remind parents to issue commands in a firm but neutral tone. Parents also should be reminded to be assertive rather than passive or aggressive. After children comply with commands, parents should praise the child by using specific labeled praise ("I like the way you listened," "Thank you for . . . the first time you were told"). Tell parents that even if they don't see an immediate effect on their child's behavior, they should continue to use their praise and attention to help their child's self-esteem and to be encouraging to their child.

CHAPTER 7

Module 7: Time Out and Privilege Removal

(Recommended Length: 1 or 2 Sessions)

Materials Needed for the Module

Forms, parent summaries, worksheets, and handouts appear in Appendix A: Client Materials, located at the end of this therapist guide. You may photocopy this material for your clients, or you may download these items from the Treatments ThatWork Web site at www.oxfordclinicalpsych.com/ADHDparenting. For an outline of this and all modules, go to Appendix B: Therapist Outlines.

Parent Materials

- Module 7 Parent Summary
- Worksheet 7.1: Looking at Connections: My Mood/Stress, Caregiving, Activities, and Thoughts
- Worksheet 7.2: Special Time and Child Behavior Record Form
- Handout 7.1: Using My CBT Skills to Help Me with Time Out

Assessment to Be Given at Every Session

- Form B: Top Problems

Home Practice Review from Module 6

During Module 6, parents learned about assertiveness and how to apply assertiveness skills to improve communication with others. Parents also learned to increase the effectiveness of parental commands and identified a few house rules to implement. Review the worksheets the parent completed tracking their Special Time, daily mood ratings, pleasant activities, and changing thoughts, as well as relaxation and assertiveness skills practice. It is important to briefly review the forms given for home practice in the previous session and check in with parents about how their practice is going with all skills covered so far. If parents used another way of tracking their practice (electronic calendar or app), you can review these as well. The following questions can be used to facilitate the home practice discussion of Module 6 skills:

Effective Commands

- *How did it go giving your child directions following the suggestions we talked about last week?*
- *What "mistakes" with giving directions did you catch?* (Make sure they give themselves credit for catching mistakes. That's the hardest part!)
- *How did your child respond to directions?* (Make sure they know it is OK if children still had a hard time following directions; giving a good direction is just the first step in helping children to learn to better follow directions.)

House Rules

- *Did you have a family meeting with your child(ren) to discuss house rules? How did that go?*
- *What rules did you decide on?*
- *Did you have opportunities to point out when your child was not following the rules and to praise when they were following the rules?*
- *Did you write the rules down and post them somewhere for your child to see?*

Assertiveness

- *How did the assertive imagery practice go? Are you becoming more clear on your boundaries (i.e., what is okay and not okay for you)?*

- *When did you use your assertiveness skills? How did others respond?*
- *Were there any situations where you noticed your use of passive or aggressive communication?*

Therapist Note

Make sure to adjust the home practice review based on what was assigned in the previous session. If topics haven't been covered yet, omit questions about that content from the home practice review. Also, if this home practice review does not include content that has been covered and assigned for home practice (e.g., if you are doing modules in a different order), make sure to expand the home practice review to include all assigned items.

Overall Module 7 Goals and Rationale

During Module 7, parents learn to use *time out from positive reinforcement* (TOR or "time out" for short) to help their child improve their ability to follow directions and rules. Children with attention-deficit/hyperactivity disorder (ADHD) benefit from parents who consistently follow through with a consequence for noncompliance and rule-breaking to reduce these child misbehaviors. Time out is effective when used *in the presence of a secure relationship and where opportunities for connection and positive reinforcement are consistently available in the home environment.*

In Modules 1 through 6, parents learned proactive and positive behavioral strategies to help their child with behavioral concerns. Parents have (1) established regular Special Time, (2) changed antecedents (schedules, effective commands, and house rules), and (3) used praise and active ignoring. Positive reinforcement is hopefully more frequent, consistent, and contingent on expected behavior.

 The ABC model of child behavior helps us understand why inappropriate behaviors are more likely to happen again when directions and rules are not enforced consistently: misbehavior continues to have positive consequences. In the following examples of the ABC model of child behavior, the parent uses a proactive parenting strategy for the antecedent but does not follow through with a limit when needed. Thus, behaviors like noncompliance and rule-breaking are positively reinforced in the absence of limit-setting. Children with ADHD benefit from the structure, consistency, and predictability of the time out consequence to reduce problem behaviors. In fact, time out is thought to help children learn to self-regulate.

The following are examples of how inappropriate behaviors are reinforced without limit-setting using the ABC model of child behavior:

- A: Effective command
- B: Child refuses to follow direction
- C: Parent does task for child or child escapes demand (negative reinforcement for both parent and child)

- A: Clear house rule (no hurting) is explained at a calm time
- B: Child breaks house rule by hitting sibling
- C: Child receives parental attention (positive reinforcement)

It is important in this module to instill hope that time out can be effective for their family even if past attempts to use time out (or other consequences) were not successful. The common challenges that families encounter when doing TOR will be addressed. In addition, you will help parents to see that their assertiveness, relaxation, and constructive thinking skills (Modules 4, 5, and 6) can help them follow through with TOR when it may have been difficult to do so previously without these skills. Children are expected to react to time out in ways that can make it hard to follow through. Parents need to be prepared to manage their own emotional experience and their child's reaction to experience the full benefits of TOR.

Specific goals for this module include:

- **Goal 1:** Provide the rationale for TOR as an effective consequence in the ABC model of child behavior.
- **Goal 2:** Teach parents how to use TOR effectively at home.
- **Goal 3:** Help parents use antecedents and TOR to improve behavior in public settings.
- **Goal 4:** Teach parents to use their assertiveness, relaxation, and self-talk skills when using TOR.

> *Goal 1: Provide the rationale for TOR as an effective*
> *consequence in the ABC model of child behavior*

In Modules 1 through 6, parents have learned many building blocks to create a therapeutic environment for their child with ADHD. These include doing a regular Special Time with their child, frequent praise for appropriate behaviors (including praise for effort), maintaining a schedule and routines, active ignoring for mild and attention-seeking misbehavior, giving effective commands, and establishing house rules. At this point, parents are likely to report observable changes in their child's behavior. *Draw the ABC model of child behavior* to show how the parents have used antecedents (daily Special Time, effective commands and house rules, schedules and routines) and consequences (praise, active ignoring) to improve their relationship with their child and the child's behavior. Choose examples of behaviors that have been addressed that are most relevant for the family. Possible examples include (1) the parent praises calm behavior and actively ignores arguing, (2) the parent praises patience and actively ignores whining, and (3) the parent praises gentle play with sibling and actively ignores mildly annoying behaviors.

Let the parent know that today you will focus on behaviors like rule-breaking, noncompliance, and/or aggression that can't be fully addressed with the strategies discussed so far. Parents have likely asked in previous sessions about what to do when these more serious behaviors occur and can't be ignored. You can say something like,

> *As we have discussed throughout this program, your attention is a very powerful reward for your child. You have been working hard to praise your child for effort and appropriate behaviors! You are also actively ignoring behaviors that are mildly annoying or attention-seeking so they are not accidentally rewarded with your attention. However, there are some behaviors that can't be ignored, like rule-breaking and noncompliance. Today we are going to talk about an effective consequence for these challenging behaviors that may be causing problems for your child in their daily routines and relationships with others.*

Ask parents what they currently do when their child does not follow directions or breaks rules. Answers may include yelling, lecturing, ignoring, reminding them of rules, threats, removing privileges, and time out. Parents may share that consequences do not seem to motivate their child or that their child's behavior gets worse when consequences are given. They may also share that they themselves are inconsistent with their use of consequences for a variety of reasons (child's reaction, parent stress, parents not on same page, etc.). Let the parent know that many families experience these difficulties when giving consequences to their child. You can say:

*Many parents have difficulty finding consequences that work for their child and family. Today you will learn how to use a consequence which (1) can be used consistently, (2) is effective in reducing problem behaviors, and (3) will help your child improve self-control. This consequence is called **time out from positive reinforcement (time out or TOR for short)**. You may have tried to use time out in the past and did not have success. You will learn today how to use time out effectively and to correct some common mistakes that families make when they attempt to use consequences. We will also talk about using the coping skills you have learned in the program (like changing your thoughts and feelings) to help you navigate some of the challenges that arise when your family begins to use time out.*

Like puzzle pieces fitting together, let parents know that time out is used in combination with the strategies they have learned in the program so far. Routines, effective commands and clear house rules, praise (for listening and following rules), and time out are used together to help their child with rule following and self-control. When TOR is done correctly, children are learning to (1) respect healthy limits, (2) cope when things are not going as expected or desired, and (3) develop self-control to reduce impulsive behaviors.

To help establish the rationale for TOR, you can remind parents that children with ADHD have a *performance deficit*, rather than a knowledge deficit. Repeated discussions about expected behavior after a child has misbehaved can be frustrating for both parents and children. You can say:

> *Children with ADHD often know what is expected but have trouble **performing** those behaviors, so responding to misbehavior with reminders and lectures does not change the behavior. It is helpful to ask yourself the question "When I do X, what does my child learn?"* [Examples: "When I lecture (or yell) after my child hits, what does my child learn?" Most parents agree that their child does not appear to learn something that positively influences future behavior. Alternatively, "When I give my child a time out for hitting, what does my child learn? My child learns that, if they want to stay in a situation with opportunities for positive interactions and privileges, rules must be followed."]

A variety of reactions occur when parents hear that you will be teaching time out. This can range from mild doubt about the effectiveness of time out to strong criticism of the use of time out when a child is having intense emotions. Make sure to (briefly) validate the parents' concerns about time out ("I can understand that you would be concerned about. . . .") and let them know that you will talk more about their concerns after you explain how time out is done in this program. You can say:

> *Many parents are unsure about the use of time out. When used in combination with the other things you have learned in this program, time out can help your child with self-control and emotion regulation. It can also be helpful for parents' emotion regulation in the most challenging*

situations with your child. In other words, by proactively having a plan
for what to do when your child breaks a house rule and practicing skills
to keep calm, it can help you avoid being reactive in emotionally charged
situations.

Goal 2: Teach parents how to use TOR effectively at home

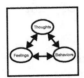

It is a process for children to learn that problem behaviors will receive a meaningful consequence each and every time they occur. These behaviors did not show up suddenly, and they will not decrease suddenly either. This may be the hardest part of the effective use of TOR: to be consistent when behavior problems are still frequent and intense. For *parent motivation*, it can be helpful to ask parents to imagine their child following directions and rules and how this would benefit their family and child. You can also ask the parents: "What will help you to cope with your child's reaction to time out as they adjust to this change?" Hopefully they will think of the cognitive-behavioral therapy (CBT) model and the skills they have practiced: helpful thinking, relaxation, assertive communication, and pleasant activities. You can tell them that, later in the session, you will return to the discussion of how their coping strategies will help them to be most successful with implementing time out.

Some of the key elements that you will teach parents to do TOR effectively include:

1. Less talking (talking is attention and attention is not part of time out!).
2. The caregiver is in charge of when time out begins and ends.
3. There is no escape from a demand (only compliance ends time out when noncompliance is the reason for time out).
4. There is a clear plan that will be followed when the child refuses to go to time out or leaves time out early.

By conveying the expectation that a plan is needed *when* (not *if!*) a child leaves time out, you are helping parents to have realistic expectations and to be adequately prepared. For children with ADHD, the use of TOR is helpful because it can be done (1) immediately, (2) briefly (after child accepts time out), and (3) there is a clear connection between *behavior* and *consequence* to help with motivation for less desirable tasks.

Explain and Model the TOR Steps (Stoplight Analogy)

It can be helpful for parents to think of time out as a three-step process, like a stop light (Barkley, 2013). As you go through each step, it is helpful to model and role-play so that parents have practice before using it with their child.

Give a Direction

The first step (**green light**) is when the parent gives their child a direction. The parent sets their child up for success by using the effective command guidelines and assertiveness skills (Module 6). After the command is given, instruct the parent to count backwards from 5 to 1 out loud to let their child know that compliance is expected right away. This can be a big change for children who are used to talking, dawdling, negotiating, or arguing after a direction is given. It is important for the parent to remain direct and firm and *only count* with no other talking. Remember, a key element to effective time out is less talking! After a few weeks, parents can begin to count silently so that their child does not wait until the parent counts down to 1 and because other adults (like teachers) will not count when compliance is necessary. To start, if the parent counts out loud, this prevents them from saying extra words (e.g., repeating the command, explaining reasons, or negotiating), and it will help the child learn that the parent plans to follow through quickly. At first, the counting serves as a helpful reminder to the child that the parent will be acting in a different way than before.

Give a Warning

If the parent counts down to 1 and their child has not started to follow the direction, the parent will say a warning: "If you don't (do what I said), then you are going to sit in the time out chair" (and point to the chair). This is like the **yellow light** in the stop light analogy. After the warning is given, the parent will count down again from 5 to 1 (out loud at first and then silently after the child is familiar with time out steps).

Time Out for Noncompliance (Red Light)

If the parent counts to 1 again and the child has not started to follow the direction, the child is now at the **red light** in the analogy. The parent will say: "You did not do what I told you to do; now you are going to the time out chair." The child is then taken quickly, calmly, and safely to the chair. When the child is sitting, the parent says: "Stay there until I say you can get up." The parent then walks away (to not give any attention) but should keep the child in view. The parent will return to the chair when the child's time out is over to see if the child is ready to follow the direction (or ready to follow the house rule).

Parents may ask about what to do if their child tries to follow the original direction after the parent has told them to go to the time out chair. It is common for children to attempt to have a "last chance" when they realize their parent intends to follow through. Tell parents that it is important for them to follow through with time out and have the child wait to follow the direction until time out is over. This will help the child to learn that dawdling is not allowed and time out cannot be escaped with this behavior (waiting until the red light to listen). Following through quickly when the time out statement is made will help the child to be very clear about what the expectation is and prevent the child from challenging this limit in the future.

Time Out for House Rules (Red Light)

In Module 6, parents identified house rules and shared these at a calm time with their child (e.g., in a family meeting). House rules are made for behaviors that are never allowed, such as no hurting people or pets. To use time out for house rule violations, parents will take their child to time out with no discussion about the behavior *and no warning*. The child is already at the red light when they break the rule so the parent only gives the time out statement: "You hit so you are going to the time out chair."

Take the Child to the Chair

Model to the parent how to take their child calmly and quickly to the time out chair. You can demonstrate walking toward the child as you say the time out statement ("You did not do what I told you to do; now you are going to the time out chair") so that the parent is in close physical proximity to their child as they say the time out statement. For younger children, show the parent how to safely carry the child to time out. For older children, you will later talk to the parent about what to do if the child refuses to go to time out and the parent is not able to take them to the chair. As long as the child is going to the chair or sitting on the chair, all behaviors are ignored. Children will react in a variety of ways including threatening, aggression, pleading, crying, and cursing. Parents need to understand the importance of continuing with the TOR steps no matter what their child is saying or doing, and not respond.

Therapist Note

If you are working with the parent of a younger child (usually age 7 or younger, depending on the child's size and parent's mobility), you will need to demonstrate how to carry a child to the timeout chair if the child is not walking to the chair with guidance. Parents should be instructed to wrap their arms around their child (under the child's armpits and across the chest). The parents should do this from behind the child (child facing away from parent) so if the child is kicking they are kicking out, not at the parent. Tell the parent they should never pull a child by their arms or drag them to timeout because that could result in an injury.

Time Out Chair and Placement

Parents should choose a sturdy chair that can be placed in a location where the child can be easy to watch. Dining rooms, kitchens, or hallways can be a good place for the time out chair. The chair should be in a safe and (ideally) boring location. Placing the chair away from walls and furniture prevents the child from kicking or grabbing things while in time out. Sometimes stairs can be in a good location for time out and the bottom step can be designated as the time out spot.

When the Child Is on the Chair

A brief TOR is sufficient for children to find it unpleasant (boring) enough to be sufficiently motivated to avoid it. Younger children need a bit less time than older children for it to be effective. A common guideline to use is no more than 1 minute per year of the child's age. After the child has sat for their time out, parents should wait for at least 5 seconds of quiet before returning to the chair. This helps the child learn that sitting quietly in the chair is a necessary condition for the parent to return to the time out chair. For example, if a 5-year-old child goes to time out (5 years old = 5-minute time out) and the child is not quiet after 5 minutes in the chair, the parent extends the time out until there are 5 seconds of quiet. If it takes 8 minutes for the child to be quiet for 5 seconds, then the time out lasts 8 minutes. Parents will often ask if they can remind their child of the need to be quiet when their child continues to cry, yell, or make other noises on the chair. Giving any attention during the time out, including reminders to be quiet, should be avoided because it will be harder for the child to learn that talking does not happen during a time out (one of the key elements shared earlier). Remind parents that their child will be calmer and quieter on the chair in the future if they wait to talk to their child.

This is a good time to emphasize that the child will learn most by *what the parent does, not what the parent says*. Why is this? Because talking during time out is attention, and any behavior that gets attention will be reinforced. Thus, when the parent talks to the child while the child is making noise in time out, the child learns that these behaviors result in parent attention. If parents wait until their child is quiet, the child learns that being quiet results in parent attention. Also, when parents wait until their child is quiet, the child is showing better regulation and readiness to return to the task or demand (or if they went into time out for breaking a house rule, to calmly re-enter the situation). Many children need a longer time out at the beginning because they have not learned to sit quietly and their emotions are intense. Help parents to understand the benefits of following through and waiting until their child is quiet before the parent returns to the chair. Remember, *too much talking is one of the key ways that time out becomes less effective*. You can say:

> *After your child has completed the number of minutes you determined for the time out, do not attempt to talk to your child until they have been quiet for at least 5 seconds. If your child is yelling or saying things to attempt to get your attention and you go to the chair at that time, those behaviors will be reinforced (more likely to happen again). If you wait*

until your child is quiet, they will learn that being quiet is necessary for you to return to the chair. Your child will learn most by what you do (waiting until they are quiet) rather than what you say (reminding them they need to be quiet). At first the time out may last much longer than a few minutes because your child is not quiet. However, your child will soon learn that staying quiet is necessary, and time outs will become shorter if you wait for quiet. Also, when your child is able to sit quietly, it indicates improved self-regulation and readiness to complete the task or rejoin the family.

Therapist Note

For parents who have a difficult time when their child is upset in the chair and feel very strongly that their child needs a reminder about sitting quietly in the chair, tell them that during their child's first time out they can tell their child ONE time: "I am not coming back to the chair until you are quiet."

The best time to remind a child to sit quietly on the chair is when the child is not in a time out. Before starting time out at home, parents are encouraged to explain the time out steps when children are calm and to tell them exactly what will happen if they get out of the chair or if they are not quiet on the chair (more information later in the module).

When the Child Is Quiet on the Chair

Next explain to parents that when they return to their child, the next step is to see if the child agrees to follow the direction. For example, if the child was told to put something away, the parent would ask, "Are you ready to put that away?" and the child must agree to do this right now. Otherwise, they will have successfully avoided doing something they did not want to do. If the child refuses, time out starts over and all of the steps are followed again (the child completes the time out minutes, the short period of quiet, and the parent asks if the child is ready to follow the direction). If the child went to time out for breaking a rule, the parent asks the child if they are ready to follow the rule. If the child does not agree to follow the house rule, a new time out begins.

When the Child Follows the Direction

Ask the parent what they should do after the child follows the direction. Hopefully they will say "praise the child for listening"! It is important that parents understand that as soon as time out is over, the child receives positive attention. The consequence has been completed, and the child is back to "time-in." If the parent stays in the past and holds on to frustration about their child's misbehavior, their child does not learn the difference between what happens when they are behaving and when they are breaking rules. When a time out is just completed, important learning occurs: children get the full benefits of attention and privileges as they follow directions and rules.

When the Child Refuses to Sit in Time Out

It is important for parents to have a clear plan of what to do when their child refuses time out. For many children it is not *if* the child refuses, but rather *when* the child refuses. If parents have reasonable expectations about this behavior, it will help them to follow through calmly and consistently. When a child leaves the time out chair (or refuses to go), the child receives one warning: "If you get out of the chair again, you will have to go to your room." Have parents practice saying this statement with a firm stance and tone. When children are refusing time out, emotions will be intensifying for both the parent and child. Parents may experience anger, guilt, or anxiety, which can impact their ability to effectively hold the limit (you will discuss this more in the next section of this module). During practice of the time out steps, encourage parents to use their assertiveness skills as needed.

When first using the child's bedroom for the time out, parents can remove toys or books or screens (otherwise the bedroom will be reinforcing!). Parents should also remove any items that may be broken or make the room unsafe (e.g., lamps, cords). If parents have concerns about being able to physically move their child to their bedroom, they may want to first practice when another adult is available to assist.

If the parent is not able to use the bedroom as a back-up for getting off the chair or refusing to go on the chair, a privilege can be taken away for a brief period of time (e.g., it is often more effective to remove a privilege for 30 minutes rather than a full day) like screen time, a toy, or time with friends. A more prolonged removal of a privilege (versus a few minutes of time out) can contribute to more misbehavior because the privilege is already gone, giving the child less incentive to act appropriately. Encourage parents to try to use the time out process as described so children receive a more immediate, brief consequence, which is more effective because children have the opportunity for "time-in" and privileges, which encourage appropriate behavior.

Another option if the child gets off the chair before time out is over is to put the child back on the chair and restart the time. The child will get some parent attention when returned to the chair so parents need to be able to follow through with a longer time out. If the use of the bedroom is an option when the child gets off the chair, make sure to emphasize the benefits of using their room to give less parental attention in the time out process.

While the Child Is on the Chair

Children will say and do many things on the chair to try to end time out or get their parent's attention. They may say they need the bathroom or that they feel sick or thirsty, say things that pull at the heartstrings ("I don't love you!"), or use inappropriate language. The most effective way to respond to these behaviors during a time out is to actively ignore them. If these behaviors result in the parent interacting with their child during time out, time out becomes less effective and these behaviors are likely to happen again in the future. A child may also stay on the chair but move (scoot) or tip the chair to test limits. If the child moves the chair the parent should give one warning ("if you move the chair again you will have to go to your room") or provide a warning describing the alternative back-up procedure ("if you move the chair again you will lose X privilege for thirty minutes") and then the behavior (tipping, moving) counts as "off the chair" if it happens again.

When a child's time out is over, they may test their parent by refusing to leave time out. If this is done, the parent should restart the time out and not engage with their child until another time out is completed.

Starting to Use Time Out at Home

When first using time out, it is recommended that a parent choose one or two situations (such as turning off a device when given a direction to do so) or a house rule (like no hurting). Because time outs may be much longer at first, it is important to avoid giving too many time outs in one day. Parents should also start using time out under usual conditions (e.g., best not to start time out on vacation or when people are visiting!). Remind parents that they have many skills to help with their child's behavior and that, when they begin time out, it is especially important to:

- maintain daily Special Time,
- praise appropriate behaviors,
- actively ignore minor misbehaviors,
- give effective commands, and
- follow household routines.

Parents should tell their child about time out during a calm time (similar to the discussion about house rules). Parents should not attempt to explain it or use it for the first time when their child is being oppositional, aggressive, or feeling very angry or upset. When their child is calm, parents can explain the importance of following directions and house rules and talk about the positive things that happen for the family and child when they do things right away and obey house rules (family gets along even better, everyone feels safe and more comfortable, more time to do fun things, etc.). The parent should then walk the child through every step of the stoplight so the child knows exactly what to expect. If the parent is starting with a house rule, they need to make sure the child knows that there will not be a warning or any discussion: when a house rule is broken, the parent will only say, "You hit so you are going to the time out chair." The parent should also explain that it important for the child to stay on the chair and to sit quietly so they can complete their time out.

Time Out with Older Children

Adaptations may be needed for older children who refuse to go to time out or for whom time out is no longer developmentally appropriate. If an older child refuses to go to time out, the parent can use delayed suspension of privileges (e.g., no computer time for the rest of the day) for refusing time out. Following through with another consequence for the time out refusal will help increase the likelihood that the child will go to time out in the future. Parents need to make sure the privilege is one the parent can fully control (e.g., access to screens) and one that parents can follow through on (e.g., a parent can't take away the privilege of going outside if the parent can't physically stop the child). Also, parents may need to extend the duration of time out for it to be effective for older children.

If there are significant concerns about the child harming someone else or themselves that interfere with the parents' ability to use consequences, more intensive evidence-based treatments such as *Multisystemic Therapy (MST)* should be considered (see http://www.mstservices.com/).

Goal 3: Help parents use antecedents and TOR to improve behavior in public settings

Parent reactions to behavior in public can be more reactive or inconsistent for a few reasons. The parent may feel anxious when others are watching their child misbehave, or the parent can feel angry for the disruption to the outing. For these reasons, parents benefit greatly from thinking ahead about what they will do when challenging behaviors happen outside the home. Again, we are trying to teach parents to be proactive versus reactive. Focusing on the antecedents before going out in public can help both parents and children. Parents can experience less stress when there is a clear plan that has been communicated to their child. Parents can also think about how to make the situation manageable for their child by considering where they are going, how long they will be there, and what activities will be most engaging for their child. When parents anticipate the behavioral problems that may occur in public and have a clear plan, their thoughts, actions, and feelings can change when challenges arise. When child behavior is anticipated and parents have a plan, they have more helpful thinking and feel more in control. You can show parents (by drawing the two models) how focusing on the Antecedents in the ABC model of child behavior before going in public can influence their experience in the CBT model. Planning ahead is self-care and can help to prevent misbehavior.

Next you will introduce how the strategies that parents have learned can be used in public settings. The Module 7 Parent Summary provides a summary of these strategies. First, parents will communicate with their child at the beginning of the trip the rules that the child is expected to follow (the Antecedent in the ABC model). Parents can stop at the entrance to the public place and establish a few simple rules that the child has had difficulty following in the past. For example, staying close to the parent, not touching things without permission, and not asking to buy things can be rules that are discussed before entering the public space. Other examples include using an inside voice, not running, and keeping feet on the ground (no climbing). The parent should ask the child to repeat back the rules to make sure they are remembered and understood.

Next, the parent determines an incentive that can be used during the trip for following the rules. Hopefully parents will say that they can use specific praises for following rules throughout the trip! The parent can purchase or bring a small treat and let the child know they will get the treat at the end of the trip if they follow the rules. Emphasize to parents that the incentive should be explained *before* entering the public place to help prevent misbehavior.

The parent will also tell the child what will happen if rules are broken or directions are not followed during the outgoing. Whenever possible, the parent should use time out to stay consistent with giving an immediate consequence for **rule-breaking** and noncompliance. Parents can think ahead of time about a good location for time out. The placement should be boring and safe. The child is aware *ahead of time* that the parent will follow through with time out if a rule is broken or the child does not follow a direction right away or after the warning. For younger children, parents can bring something small like a piece of paper or placemat to put on the floor to designate the time out spot.

An important antecedent for appropriate behavior in public is planning ahead for activities during the outing. Helping the child to engage in an activity is an antecedent that helps to prevent misbehavior. Examples of antecedents include looking for items at the grocery store or crossing things off the grocery list, helping to carry things or push the cart, or playing a game like "I Spy," when possible.

Time Out in Public

Giving clear expectations before entering a public setting, offering a reward at the end of the outing (or at intervals during the outing if helpful), and praising cooperation throughout the outing will help to prevent misbehavior. However, if a rule is broken or the child does not follow a direction after the time out warning is given, the parent will need to follow through with time out. Children benefit from the consistency and predictability of the time out consequence when it is used across contexts.

Parents should identify a place for time out that is safe and boring in the public space. The time out interval can be shortened in public (to about half the duration of time out used at home) because children are usually more motivated to avoid time out in public when others are watching and they are missing out on possible fun activities. For safety, the parent should remain close to the child but make sure not to give the child any attention. To end the time out in public, the parent should follow the same steps they use at home, including several moments of quiet and the child agreeing to follow the direction. If the child leaves time out early, the child should return to the time out spot and be given a warning ("If you leave time out again before I say you can, then. . . ."). Options for consequences for leaving time out in public include removing a privilege, ending the trip, or doing a time out in the car. The time out in the car can be done with the child sitting in the back seat and the parent sitting in the front seat or the parent can stand next to the car (carefully monitoring the child to make sure the child is safe). A time out in the car should only be used when the weather is appropriate and there are no safety concerns.

Emphasize to parents that the use of clear expectations before entering a public space, the use of praise and rewards, the use of activities during the outing to engage the child, and the child knowing that time out can happen in public often prevent misbehavior and the need to follow through with time out.

Goal 4: Teach parents to use their assertiveness, relaxation, and self-talk skills when using TOR

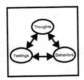

Ask parents to describe their experience when they need to give their child a consequence for not following directions or **rule-breaking**. Use the CBT model to identify patterns of thoughts, feelings, and actions (or urges) that occur when the parent needs to give their child a consequence. What thoughts do they have about their child and themselves? What thoughts do they have about their life, partner, or future when they are in a challenging moment with their child? Remind parents that their strong reactions to their child's misbehavior or their child's emotional reactions to limit setting are related to thoughts that parents and children have in these difficult situations. If the parent thinks, "I am responsible for my child's feelings" or "My child can't handle this," they may try to protect their child from discomfort. If they think, "My child is doing this on purpose," they may respond harshly or escalate to more severe punishments. If they think, "My partner doesn't support me" or "Nothing works," they may give up and not follow through. On the other hand, if the parent thinks, "My child has difficulty in these types of situations and needs help to stay in control," their reactions will be more supportive. With their knowledge of the CBT model, parents can identify helpful thoughts (e.g., "I can follow through with this reasonable limit") and healthy behaviors (e.g., relaxation practice, getting sufficient sleep) that will help them to stay calm and follow through.

You can assist parents in developing a coping plan that will support them in their use of TOR this week. This plan should include coping skills to use before and during the TOR steps with their child. Use Handout 7.1: Using My CBT Skills to Help Me with Time Out to help guide the discussion.

Coping Skills for Parents to Use Before Using the TOR Steps

- *Assertiveness skills*: Parents can let other caregivers know about their need for support. Do tasks need to be delegated so the parent has more time to follow through with time out, or does the schedule need to be changed to allow the parent time to follow through, or is more physical or emotional support needed by others so that they are available to help the parent follow through?
- *Pleasant activities*: Remind parents that when they commit to pleasant and self-care activities to reduce overall stress levels and

improve mood, this helps them with difficult parenting situations. Checking in with parents on their pleasant activity scheduling when starting time out reinforces the connection between their own well-being and their parenting.

- *Relaxation skills*: The more parents practice relaxation skills outside of challenging situations with their children, the easier it will be for parents to use these skills in more stressful situations.
- *Mindfulness*: When parents practice mindfulness throughout the day, it improves their ability to use mindfulness in challenging situations with their children. Parents can choose a task each day during which to practice mindfulness (e.g., brushing teeth, walking up the stairs, drinking tea) so they strengthen the ability to stay in the present moment during the time out steps.
- *Helpful thinking/self-talk skills*: Parents can identify and review helpful thoughts each morning to be able to use self-talk in challenging parenting situations. For example, thoughts such as, "My child needs to learn to deal with their anger without aggression. I can help them learn to do this by following through with the house rule of no hitting" can help parents to remember that time out is a way of supporting their child. Examples of helpful thoughts when the parent needs to follow through with a time out in public include, "Others are often understanding," and "This will get easier as my child learns that I will follow through each time." Suggest that parents write helpful thoughts on notecards or in their mobile phone notes so they can look at them during calm times and during a time out (see later discussion).

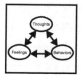

Coping Skills for Parents to Use When They Give Child a Time Out

- *Assertiveness skills*: Parents should remember to act quickly when their child is noncompliant or breaks a house rule. If there are many reminders or arguing or negotiating, there is more time for frustration to build for both parent and child. Assertiveness allows the parent to feel confident in following through quickly and calmly even when their child is feeling very upset.
- *Relaxation skills*: Parents can use relaxation skills to feel better during the time out steps. For example, when the child is on the chair or in

their room, the parent can take calming breaths. Before parents give the time out warning, they can quickly relax their muscles.

- *Mindfulness*: Parents can use mindfulness to stay in the present moment without judgment of themselves or their child. Mindfulness helps parents to *respond rather than react* in stressful situations because they are aware of their experience.
- *Helpful thinking/self-talk skills*: Parents should remember to refer to their helpful thoughts, which they have previously identified, to help them stay calm and follow through with time out. Again, having a notecard ready and available with coping statements, such as, "One way I show my love for my child is calmly setting limits," and "I can help my child to learn that this behavior is not okay." Remind parents that it is natural to feel anxious, angry, or upset when they are in a challenging parenting situation, and it is helpful to have reminders of things to say to themselves in the moment to stay calm.
- *Delayed response*: If parents are too angry or anxious to calmly respond to their child, they can briefly walk away until they can calmly follow through with the time out steps. Parents are models for their children, and how parents handle their own reactions is very important for children to learn how to manage their own emotions!

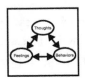 Before ending the session, make sure to ask about any parental concerns that remain about the use of TOR. Use motivational interviewing, CBT, and problem-solving techniques to address their concerns. If parents focus on negative experiences with using time out in the past, ask them how the information they learned today might change the way they approach time out now. You can share that parents should notice a difference when they use time out calmly and quickly rather than after emotions have escalated or inconsistently. If parents continue to question time out as an appropriate consequence for their child, provide more psychoeducation about the benefits of structure and limit-setting for children with ADHD when they are used in combination with the strategies discussed in other modules. You can ask more about current strategies for enforcing limits and how effective they are.

Last, make sure that concerns about other caregivers interfering with the use of the time out consequence are addressed. For example, others may believe that the child's behavior is "normal" and doesn't require consequences such as time out. Or the parents may have collectivist values and be highly influenced by criticism of time out by other family members. Some family members may think that serious child misbehavior warrants physical punishment. Assist the parent with identifying who needs more information about the child's needs and treatment approach, what specific information others need, and how that information can be delivered most effectively to others (share handouts, schedule a call with you, schedule a one-on-one conversation at a calm time, etc.).

Home Practice

At the end of each session, distribute the Parent Module Summary and reinforce the fact that the information discussed today will now be practiced at home. Home practice for this module includes

- Completing Worksheet 7.1: Looking at Connections: My Mood/Stress, Caregiving, Activities, and Thoughts
- Completing Worksheet 7.2: Special Time and Child Behavior Record Form

You should emphasize to the parent that this is an especially important week to continue with Special Time. It will help to balance out the focus on consequences this week. Parents should also plan to complete the time out procedure focusing on 1–2 behaviors or house rules. Make sure parents set up the chair beforehand and explain to their child what will happen if a direction is not followed or a house rule is broken. Point out that there is a new column on Worksheet 7.2: Special Time and Child Behavior Record Form to track whether a child went to time out and briefly write about how it went.

CHAPTER 8

Module 8: Working Effectively with the Schools

(Recommended Length: 2 or 3 Sessions)

Therapist Note

This module should be delivered during or immediately preceding the school year. If the child is having a great deal of difficulty with school behavior, this module can come earlier in the program, but ideally parents will have the foundational behavioral and cognitive-behavioral therapy (CBT) skills before this module is delivered.

Materials Needed for the Module

Forms, parent summaries, worksheets, and handouts appear in Appendix A: Client Materials, located at the end of this therapist guide. You may photocopy this material for your clients, or you may download these items from the Treatments ThatWork web site at www.oxfordclinicalpsych.com/ ADHDparenting. For an outline of this and all modules, go to Appendix B: Therapist Outlines.

Parent Materials

- Module 8 Parent Summary
- Worksheet 8.1: Daily Report Card
- Worksheet 8.2: Social Skills and Assertiveness
- Worksheet 8.3: Looking at Connections: My Mood/Stress, Caregiving, Activities, and Thoughts

- Worksheet 8.4: Special Time and Child Behavior Record Form
- Handout 8.1: Sample Daily Report Card

Assessment to Be Given at Every Session

- Form B: Top Problems

Home Practice Review from Module 7

In Module 7, parents learned to use time out from positive reinforcement (TOR) to help their child improve their ability to follow directions and rules. Review the home practice worksheets from last session and resolve any problems the parents may be having in their use of the time out procedure and/or privilege removal. Spend time going through examples to ensure that parents understand the concepts and are using these procedures correctly. As they provide examples, reiterate concepts from the previous session (time out away from reinforcing activities; minimizing attention to the child while in time out, etc.). You can ask:

- *How did time out seem to work? Where did you do it? For what behaviors did your child receive a time out?*
- *What were your thoughts and feelings during your child's time out? Did you use any relaxation or mindfulness strategies to keep calm?*

Problem-solve with parents regarding problems/issues that came up. Time out is a difficult skill so it is important to spend adequate time to work out any problems that arose. If time allows, check in with parents about their other home practice (Special Time, pleasant activities, etc.). Maintaining these positive strategies will be very important during this time to make "time in" as reinforcing as possible.

Therapist Note

Make sure to adjust the home practice review based on what was assigned in the previous session. If topics haven't been covered yet, omit questions about that content from the home practice review.

Also, if this home practice review does not include content that has been covered and assigned for home practice (e.g., if you are doing modules in a different order), make sure to expand the home practice review to include all assigned items.

Overall Module 8 Goals and Rationale

During Module 8, parents learn the importance of advocating for their children's educational needs by developing and maintaining a collaborative working relationship with the school. Some parents (for a variety of reasons) are hesitant to talk to the school and ask for what they need, whereas others may be demanding and/or even aggressive in their requests. (Refer to Module 6 for the passive-assertive-aggressive continuum.) The most effective outcomes tend to come when parent(s) and school *collaboratively* work together toward the common goal of helping the child succeed.

To be the most effective *advocate* for the child, parents must understand their educational rights. Parents should also be familiar with **evidence-based strategies** for addressing academic productivity and behavior management in the classroom so that they know what to ask for. Examples include the daily report card (DRC), maintaining consistent routines and structure, classroom rules, breaking down long-term assignments into smaller components with intermediate deadlines, and organizational skills training. These behavioral approaches are very similar to those the parents have been learning in this program.

Parents may assume that recommendations and accommodations suggested by the school are evidence-based (meaning there is well-designed research supporting their efficacy), when in fact research suggests that many supports and accommodations provided on Individual Education Plans (IEPs) and 504 Plans are unfortunately not evidence-based. Parents therefore need to be prepared to educate others about what is effective.

A subset of parents will need support to appropriately assert themselves in this context, refraining from being either too passive or too aggressive (Module 6). Many parents will also need to be reminded to *express gratitude* (and to use other social skills) toward teachers and school staff who demonstrate a commitment to helping their child.

A subset of parents will also need support with *keeping organized records* of their children's psychological evaluations, report cards, discipline reports, emails from teachers, and so on to make a convincing argument for the need for or refinement of special services. Such organization will also be essential as they prepare for school (e.g., IEP, 504 Plan) meetings.

Specific goals for this module include

- **Goal 1:** Teach parents about the importance of establishing and maintaining a collaborative working relationship with the school.
- **Goal 2:** Work with the parents to understand the child's educational rights so that they can effectively advocate for their child.
- **Goal 3:** Familiarize the parent with evidence-based approaches to classroom behavior management.
- **Goal 4:** Introduce social, assertiveness, and organizational skills that will help parents be most effective in working with their child's school.

Module 8 Content (Divided by Goals)

> *Goal 1: Teach parents about the importance of establishing and maintaining a collaborative working relationship with the school*

By the time parents make their way to therapy, often the relationship between parents and the school has become extremely negative. Each side may blame the other for what they have or have not done to support the student academically and behaviorally. Perhaps the school has not done things in the past to support the student, or the parent has not done their part to support the child's academics at home—and as a result, resentment has built over time. A collaborative, working relationship between parents and the school can impact how effectively and efficiently the child can get what they need in the school setting. You can say something like,

Imagine getting a call from someone at work who has not been very nice to you or appreciative of you in the past, someone who has blamed you for negative things that have happened and/or who is demanding you do

something without any sense of how much work that will place on you and/or who is not acknowledging all the work you have already done. Now imagine receiving a request from someone you view as a collaborator, who listens to and values your input, asks for your impressions, and demonstrates a desire to work together toward a common goal. Receiving a call from the first person may feel immediately dreadful, but a call from the second person can feel quite productive and good if you both have concerns and want to work together on a solution.

Parents and teachers both fundamentally want what is best for the child, and working together is essential for reaching this goal. Simple things like expressing appreciation, being willing to work with the teacher and acknowledging the teacher's experience/expertise in the classroom can be helpful to building a healthy foundation for the behavioral work that will ensue.

> **Goal 2: Work with the parent to understand the child's educational rights so that they can effectively advocate for their child**

Children with attention-deficit/hyperactivity disorder (ADHD) may be deemed eligible for accommodations under Section 504 of the Rehabilitation Act of 1973 (called Section 504) or the Individuals with Disabilities Education Act (IDEA). The difference between these two is laid out here:

https://chadd.org/for-parents/educational-rights/

Whether the child is eligible for accommodations under Section 504 versus an IEP under IDEA depends on the extent to which ADHD affects the child's academic progress and social behavior in the classroom. Children with ADHD *and* a learning disability or autism spectrum disorder are automatically eligible for an IEP, but those without these comorbidities must evidence clear impairments academically and/or severe behavioral issues in the classroom to qualify for an IEP. In other words, ADHD on its own is not sufficient to warrant an IEP, but ADHD may fall under the "other health impaired (OHI)" category if academic impacts are severe enough to warrant this. Section 504 is another (somewhat easier) way to obtain accommodations for children with ADHD to ensure accessibility to education (similar to ramps allowing wheelchair access for people with a physical disability). However, the legal "teeth" behind an IEP are much stronger than for the 504.

Almost half of students with ADHD in the United States do not have either an IEP or 504 Plan (DuPaul, Chronis-Tuscano, Danielson, & Visser, 2019). Research examining who does and does not get services for ADHD in the schools found that adolescents with ADHD as well as children and adolescents from lower income, non–English-speaking families are less likely to get school services (DuPaul et al., 2019). It is likely that lower income and non–English-speaking parents are less informed about their children's rights, feel less comfortable advocating for their children, and do not know what to ask for. As the therapist, an important role you play is helping parents to learn their rights and to advocate for what their child needs to be successful.

If a parent wishes to have their child's need for a 504 Plan or IEP evaluated by the school district, they should prepare a dated letter laying out their specific concerns, with accompanying documentation (e.g., report cards, emails or notes from the teacher, outside evaluation reports). A template for this letter can be found at https://chadd.org/for-parents/educational-rights/. There are laws governing how quickly the school district needs to respond to this request, as well as other procedural aspects (some of which vary by state).

Additionally, if a child has an IEP or 504 Plan that is not being implemented as documented, or if the child is continuing to struggle academically despite their accommodations, the parent can request a meeting. All correspondence should be in writing (or followed up in writing) and letters should be dated. Knowing one's rights is very important to ensuring that the child is making steady academic progress and getting the help they need. In other words, in order to be an effective advocate for their children, parents need to be informed.

School districts vary greatly in their responsiveness to a child's need for educational accommodations, and, while most school districts want what is best for their students, there are sometimes instances where the school is unwilling to adequately address the parents' concerns. The National Disability Rights Network is the largest provider of legally based advocacy services to people with disabilities in the United States. Information about services available in each state can be found at http://www.ndrn.org/en/ndrn-member-agencies.html.

Behavioral interventions like the ones described in this parenting program are considered an "evidence-based treatment" for ADHD (meaning there is well-designed research supporting their efficacy). Because ADHD symptoms are generally present both at home and school, interventions need to be delivered in both settings to be most effective. This includes antecedents such as consistent classroom structure, routines, and posted classroom rules, as well as consequences such as labeled praise, rewards, time out, and removal of privileges. Accommodations can be selected based on the child's areas of challenge (impulsivity, distractibility, disorganization) and what is motivating for the child. Accommodations can include a range of supports, including preferential seating, assignment modifications, assistance with note taking, extra materials (a set of books for home and school), schedule changes, organizational assistance (e.g., teacher checks agenda book, assists with chunking assignments), planned breaks, changes to the delivery of instruction, and much more!

In addition, the DRC (Iznardo, Rogers, Volpe, Labelle, & Robaey, 2017; Pyle & Fabiano, 2017) is an evidence-based tool that allows for regular school–home communication about the most pressing behaviors that are impeding the child's success in the classroom (academically, behaviorally, and socially). Often, parents are not aware of how the child is doing until months have passed, being informed only at parent–teacher conferences or when something serious has happened and the teacher or school administrator calls the parent. The DRC allows for regular communication about the child's progress and specific problem areas. When backed with rewards for each goal met, the DRC is also an effective way to change child behavior. Give Worksheet 8.1: Daily Report Card to the parent as well as Handout 8.1, which is an example of a completed DRC.

Parent Involvement in Consultation Meetings with the School

In some cases, you may consult directly with the school (involving the parents in most meetings in order to model effective communication and collaboration with the school) to set up the DRC. The goal is for the parent to be able to eventually take over these communications, preparing for a time when the family is no longer in therapy. In the case of higher functioning parents, you may be able to coach the parent to take on this role more independently from the get-go with your help and preparation.

Daily Report Card

Some teachers are already using some form of a DRC (sometimes referred to as a *school–home note*). When that is the case, it is often better to begin there and consult with the teacher to make the system more effective rather than to disregard their system in favor of a brand new one. This will not help rapport! Consistent with the goal of building/ maintaining a good relationship with the school, it is important in these communications for parents to maintain a pleasant attitude, acknowledging the teachers' use of effective behavioral strategies and dedication to the welfare of the child.

You may have to address the use of strategies that are not evidence-based, such as weighted vests, fidget spinners, or stability balls. Sometimes these items can be more distracting or draw unwanted attention and increase anxiety for children with ADHD. Occupational therapy interventions are often implemented for children with ADHD without benefit (Graziano, Garcia, & Landis, 2018; Macphee et al., 2019), and you may need to share information with the teacher about the evidence-based treatments that improve focus and regulation. Motivational interviewing (MI) can be helpful here in asking permission to share this information (see Introduction).

A very helpful step-by-step guide for setting up a DRC can be found at https://ccf.fiu.edu/_assets/pdfs/how_to_establish_a_school_drc.pdf. This guide can be used as an extra resource and also can be shared with school staff.

The first step in developing a DRC is to identify the 2–4 most important behaviors that need to change to help the child be more successful in school. Identifying these behaviors involves input from the teacher. Behaviors should be defined as *specifically* as possible (as in the ABC model) and should be *observable*. "Behaving" or "being good" are not specific enough and are difficult to evaluate objectively, especially across different teachers. Instead, "listen the first time," "raise your hand before speaking in class," and "not interrupting" are more appropriate DRC targets.

The second step (once you have decided upon target behaviors) is *goal setting* based on how the child is currently performing. For example, if a child is only completing 10% of their classwork, it would not be reasonable to expect them to complete 100% of their classwork. We often use the analogy of expecting someone to run a marathon if they cannot even run around the block. That would not be fair! A good rule of thumb is to set a goal that the child can achieve 75–80% of the time, and then gradually shape that goal to the desired endpoint as the child experiences increasing success.

The DRC can be broken down by morning/afternoon or by subject (if the teacher is willing to do so) to allow the child to "restart" after each period. This can also provide valuable information about the specific context(s) in which the child is having difficulty, which may be related to class structure, course content, time of day, etc. (these are all antecedents!).

The DRC can be an effective tool for changing child behavior if it is accompanied by rewards for goal attainment. *Reward systems* accompanying the DRC will take into account each and every success and not require perfection. After all, each DRC goal met is an achievement in an area that is difficult for the child. It is helpful to frame it this way to parents who may be disappointed to see only 25% of goals met. Rewards can take the form of privileges in time increments (e.g., 5 minutes of screen time for every "yes" [see Handout 8.1: Sample Daily Report Card], special privileges like being line leader or choosing the meal) and should be paired with ample labeled praise. Rewards can be delivered by the school, parents, or some combination. School-based rewards have the ability to be more immediate but place more demands on the teacher. Home-based rewards are somewhat delayed but send the message that the school and home are working together and on the same page.

Keeping with our attempts to remain positive in our thinking, parents should be encouraged to respond to the child's every success with a great deal of praise (see Module 4) and to limit negative responses to unmet goals (easier said than done!). Instead, parents should be instructed to remain calm and take a problem-solving approach with the child, conveying confidence that the child can meet their goals tomorrow.

If the child has an IEP or 504 Plan, it can be helpful to include the DRC on that plan. This will formalize the use of a DRC rather than leaving it up to the individual teacher and can ensure that the DRC is carried out. In other words, if the DRC is included on an IEP or 504 Plan, then *by law* the school has to implement it.

> *Goal 4: Introduce social, assertiveness, and organizational skills that will help parents be most effective in working with their child's school*

Social Skills

Knowing that their child is having difficulty in school can be very upsetting for parents. This is a natural reaction on the part of parents who hate to see their child struggling. Sometimes when people feel stressed or upset, it affects their social skills (even if they are someone who usually possesses good social skills). Here are some examples of how our social skills may be disrupted when we are upset:

- *We may not attend social, school, or community activities or be less social when we do go.* Being a presence in the school when it is feasible for the family (e.g., volunteering, attending school events) is important for parents' relationship-building with the school staff and teachers. School personnel may be more willing to help parents who are more involved with the school because they see parents putting an effort into their child's education. In other words, schools may be more willing to help parents they see "giving back."
- *We often do not pay attention to the feelings or perspectives of others when we are feeling stressed or upset.* This sometimes means that we don't ask other people questions about how they are doing or what they are thinking. We may be less likely to listen carefully when they are talking. This may prevent parents from seeing the teacher's perspective or acknowledging the efforts the teacher has made with the child, regardless of whether those efforts were successful.

- *When we are stressed, we may be more sensitive to feeling ignored or rejected.* Parents may be more prone to getting upset by an unanswered email or phone call without realizing that teachers receive many messages and may not be able to respond during a busy school day.
- *Sometimes when we feel stressed or upset, we may behave more aggressively.* We may anger more easily and react more explosively. This will most certainly have a negative impact on the parent–teacher relationship. Importantly, this will interfere with effective communication and likely have a negative impact on the success of a collaborative home–school behavior program.

You can say something like,

> *You can think about your own levels of stress about your child's behavior at school and how that might influence your social skills. You can ask yourself, "How do I appear to others when I am stressed or upset?" Sometimes it is also helpful to ask people you are close to (and trust!) for honest feedback on how you behave when you are upset or stressed. It's important to be open to that feedback and stay calm, remembering they have your best interests in mind and want to help.*
>
> *Certain social skills lead to more positive responses from others:*
>
> - *Smiling/laughing*
> - *Complimenting others when appropriate*
> - *Fully listening when someone is talking to you*
> - *Expressing agreement when you agree*
> - *Sharing what you have in common (for example, shared goals)*
> - *Giving an opinion in a non-threatening way*
> - *Expressing appreciation for what the other person has done for you or your child*
>
> *By using good social skills when you interact with your child's school, you can build a positive foundation from which to make requests regarding extra assistance related to your child's learning and behavior problems.*

It may be helpful to introduce the concept of "mindful emailing." In order to use our social skills, we may need to wait until intense emotions pass. It is usually better to wait to respond than to send an emotionally reactive email. For email communication, we recommend asking yourself, "Would I say this in person?" and check on the tone of your email. You can say something like,

Imagine the person you are sending it to and how you want them to receive the information (not passive or aggressive). Give yourself some time (e.g., 24 hours) if you are feeling very angry or anxious and re-read the email before sending it.

Therapist Note

Of course, there will be some times when the parents do everything right and they still are met with opposition from the school. In these instances, a carefully thought-out plan developed with your help will be necessary. It will also be important to praise parents for their efforts and encourage them to persist in advocating for their child. If the school is legitimately not meeting the child's needs, parents may wish to consult with a special education lawyer or advocate.

Assertiveness Skills

Working effectively with the school and advocating for a child's educational rights also requires the parent to be *assertive* (see Module 6). Assertiveness means letting others know what you feel and need without acting angry or pushy or like a bully (which would be defined as aggressive). Assertive people can feel confident in sharing what they think and can stick up for themselves and their children without coming off as aggressive.

When we feel upset, we may be less assertive and may not say what we are thinking or stick up for ourselves. Alternatively, we may make demands without using our social skills and may even reach the point of being aggressive—which rarely gets parents very far when working with the schools. Rather, fostering an open, collaborative relationship with regular parent–teacher communication sets the foundation for the school to want to help the child.

Referring back to Figure 6.1, you can draw a continuum on the board, with passive on one end and aggressive on the other. Write examples on the board for each spot on the continuum, particularly related to interactions with the school. Ask parents for suggestions of each type of communication using school examples relevant to them.

In situations in which you have a hard time being assertive, you can practice imagining yourself being assertive and what you would say/do. [You can refer to their practice in Module 6 if they did this.] *This practicing makes it easier to act assertively when the situation comes up. For example, if you have a hard time making a request for someone to do something for your child, imagine yourself making a request confidently and nicely. Imagine these situations having positive outcomes. Then imagine the person responding in a difficult way and how you would handle that assertively to show yourself that you are capable of handling challenging reactions! Remember to also incorporate helpful social skills in your imaginal practice.* [Some parents will benefit from a role-play of talking to the teacher or sharing at a school meeting so they can build confidence in their ability to respond skillfully during times of stress.]

Give the parent Worksheet 8.2: Social Skills and Assertiveness and complete the Assertiveness section as an in-session activity.

Organizational Skills

Being an effective advocate for one's child means being *informed* (e.g., about available services and special education process) and *prepared* with documentation, well-thought-out questions, etc. Being an advocate for one's child's educational needs also requires parents' active involvement in formal 504 or IEP meetings. Such participation requires a great deal of organization and planning on the part of the parent, which can be a struggle for some, such as parents with their own ADHD symptoms/ executive functioning deficits. Working with parents to develop a *file system* for documentation related to their child's academic progress is essential to effective advocacy. In other words, report cards, discipline records, teacher communication (notes, emails), testing/evaluation reports, and should all be kept together in one place. Parents may prefer to have a file with paper copies of these documents or an electronic folder on their computer with scanned copies of these documents. You can help the parent set up an organizational system that is the best fit for them and easy for them to maintain.

Moreover, parents should *actively participate* in all meetings related to a child's IEP or 504 Plan. Discuss ways for the parents to prepare in advance, including bringing written questions and identifying support people (psychologist/therapist, pediatrician, friend/family member, or a parent advocate) to help provide information, take notes, and be there with the parent. Parents should be provided with a copy of the Plan to review before the meeting and should prepare by reviewing the IEP or 504 Plan with trusted professionals (even if the professionals cannot be present at the meeting). Parents should refrain from signing the 504 Plan or IEP if there are outstanding/unresolved concerns or issues. Additional tips for an effective IEP/504 meeting can be found here: https://www.psychologytoday.com/us/blog/joyful-parenting/201601/10-ways-make-the-most-childs-iep-meeting. Parents' use of self-care (e.g., sleep, relaxation, helpful thinking) and social and assertiveness skills (as noted previously) can be helpful in maintaining composure during the meeting itself.

> **Group Options:** Here are a few questions to jump-start group discussion:
>
> - *What are some things you do to build or maintain a positive working relationship with your child's school?*
> - *Can a few people share what they notice about their social behavior when they are stressed or upset? How do you think this plays out in your interactions with your child's school?*
> - *Is anyone willing to share a situation in which they had to be assertive with the school and how it went? What did you do to prepare in advance?*

Home Practice

At the end of each session, distribute the Parent Module Summary and reinforce the fact that the information discussed today will now be practiced at home. Home practice for this module includes:

- Taking action steps toward the school-related goal (discussed later)
- Completing Worksheet 8.3: Looking at Connections: My Mood/Stress, Caregiving, Activities, and Thoughts
- Completing Worksheet 8.4: Special Time and Child Behavior Record Form

Action Steps

Ask parents to choose a school-related goal based on the information discussed today and identify *action steps* toward that goal. Parents will come to session with a variety of concerns and experiences related to working with their child's teacher/school. Some parents may have a very good working relationship with the teacher and school staff, a solid 504 Plan or IEP, and minimal concerns about the child's school functioning. Others will have strained relationships with the teacher/school, no formal educational plan for accommodations, and significant concerns about their child's functioning at school. Based on the information gathered today, help the parent to define a feasible goal and action steps. For parents struggling with using social and assertiveness skills with their child's school, you can also assign home practice of using imagery to build confidence with these skills. Based on the family's goals and needs, you can provide more education by recommending specific resources listed at the end of this module.

Examples of Goals

1. Request an evaluation for a 504 Plan or IEP eligibility.
2. Establish a DRC.
3. Develop an organizational system for important school information.
4. Share current concerns with child's teacher in a collaborative, positive, and assertive way.
5. Prepare for a school meeting by writing questions and identifying support people.
6. Give positive feedback to the teacher for support and the use of effective strategies.
7. Join an activity at the child's school. Volunteer if parent is able.

Additional Resources

Websites, books, and additional handouts may be helpful to make sure the parent receives the education and guidance they need to pursue support for their child at school.

- Websites:

  https://ccf.fiu.edu/_assets/pdfs/how_to_establish_a_school_drc.pdf

  www.understood.org

  www.chadd.org

  https://www.psychologytoday.com/us/blog/joyful-parenting/201601/10-ways-make-the-most-childs-iep-meeting

- Books:

  Interventions for Disruptive Behaviors: Reducing Problems and Building Skills, by Gregory Fabiano (2016).

  All About ADHD: The Complete Practical Guide for Classroom Teachers (2nd ed.), by Linda Pfiffner (2011).

CHAPTER 9

Module 9: Emotion Coaching

(Recommended Length: 1 or 2 Sessions)

Materials Needed for the Module

Forms, parent summaries, worksheets, and handouts appear in Appendix A: Client Materials, located at the end of this therapist guide. You may photocopy this material for your clients, or you may download these items from the Treatments That Work web site at www.oxfordclinicalpsych.com/ADHDparenting. For an outline of this and all modules, go to Appendix B: Therapist Outlines.

Parent Materials

- Module 9 Parent Summary
- Worksheet 9.1: Looking at Connections: My Mood/Stress, Caregiving, Activities, and Thoughts
- Worksheet 9.2: Special Time and Child Behavior Record Form
- Handout 9.1: Child Emotion List
- Handout 9.2: Emotion Coaching
- Handout 9.3: Emotion Coaching and Misbehavior

Assessment to Be Given at Every Session

- Form B: Top Problems

Home Practice Review from Module 8

During Module 8, parents learned the importance of advocating for their children's educational needs by developing and maintaining a collaborative working relationship with the school. Parents learned about daily report cards as well as assertiveness, social, and organizational skills that will help them be more effective in working with their child's school. Parents are still early on in their use of the time out consequence so remember to ask how this is going and address any questions or concerns. In addition, emphasizing self-care is important as the parents work hard to implement new child behavior-management strategies. You can use some of the following questions to facilitate the home practice review:

- *Have you had any communication with your child's school since we met and if so, how did it go? What assertiveness, social, or organizational skills did you need to use in your interactions with the school?*
- *Have you had a chance to take any action steps that we identified (request for 504 eligibility, contacting teacher about Daily Report Card, etc.)? (if applicable)*
- *How many times did your child go to time out since your last session? For what behaviors did they receive a time out? How often did you have to give the time out warning after a command (the yellow light step)?*
- *Was there at least one thing you were able to do to take care of yourself or "charge your battery" this week?*

Problem-solve with parents regarding issues that came up regarding the school-related goal. If time allows, check in with parents about their other home practice (Special Time, relaxation, etc.) based on the individual family's needs.

Therapist Note

Make sure to adjust the home practice review based on what was assigned in the previous session. If topics haven't been covered yet, omit questions about that content from the home practice review. Also, if this home practice review does not include content that has been covered and given for home practice (e.g., if you are doing modules in a different order), make sure to expand the home practice review to include all relevant items.

Overall Module 9 Goals and Rationale

During Module 9, parents will be introduced to the concept of children's emotion development and the importance of parents helping their children with attention-deficit/hyperactivity disorder (ADHD) to handle strong emotions effectively (and without acting out!).

Parents are the child's first teachers for how to regulate (or manage) their emotions. In addition to this, parents serve the role of "external regulator" for their children (Gottman & Declaire, 1998). As we have mentioned throughout this book, many children with ADHD are far more sensitive to their environments. Often they will look to their parents for signs of how to react to a situation or stressor. The intensity and manner in which the parent responds set the stage for how the child learns to respond. The goal is for parents to stay calm and collected, *modeling* effective emotion regulation for their child during periods of stress.

In addition, young children with ADHD receive a high level of negative feedback from both adults and peers in their environment. It is easy for others to forget the biological basis of their impairments and send them messages that communicate that they are seen as lazy or mean-spirited or that they should "know better." Many parents have expressed frustration when others minimize the influence of ADHD on the child's behavioral and emotional regulation and when others have the same expectations they would have for neurotypical peers. Parents can also fall into this trap themselves of having expectations that do not account for the child's ADHD-related impairments. These negative messages from others can influence the child's self-concept (how they feel about themselves). When parents learn to be emotion coaches, they are more likely to consider the child's impairments without judgment and decrease critical or invalidating responses.

The goal is to send the message to the child that we all experience emotions (both pleasant and unpleasant) and that even negative or unpleasant emotions are OK. They are indeed normal! By sending this message, parents convey that they are providing a safe space for the child to express their emotions. By serving as the child's "emotion coach" and labeling emotions, the child also learns "emotion language" so that acting out in response to emotions is not necessary to express how they are feeling.

Parent emotion coaching skills consist of

- Being *aware* of the child's emotions and triggers.
- *Validating* and *tolerating* the child's emotions.

- Using *emotion descriptions* about how the child is feeling and why.
- *Setting limits* while building *problem-solving* and *self-regulation* skills.
- Being aware of one's own reaction and regulating emotions to convey calm and support.

 You can refer to the book by Gottman and Declaire (1998) for additional reading on parent emotion coaching and the development of emotion regulation skills.

This skill of parent emotion coaching is important not only now, but also as the child moves into adolescence. By setting the foundation as being someone to with whom the child can safely express emotions, during adolescence they will be more likely to share feelings and experiences with their parent(s)—which is critically important during the high-risk teenage years when youth experience an uptick in depression, anxiety, and overall emotionality and may begin to experiment with alcohol and substances. In other words, if parents take time to attend to their child's emotions when they are young (even in relation to small things), their children will be more likely to share their emotions in relation to more serious issues in the future.

Specific goals for this module include

- **Goal 1:** Parents will come to understand their role as the child's emotion regulation model and coach.
- **Goal 2:** Help parents become more aware of and attentive to their children's emotions.
- **Goal 3:** Teach parents to (1) validate, (2) tolerate, and (3) label their children's emotions.
- **Goal 4:** Help parents discriminate between times when they should use emotion coaching versus behavioral consequences (e.g., time out, ignoring).

Module 9 Content (Divided by Goals)

Goal 1: Parents will come to understand their role as the child's emotion regulation model and coach

To introduce parents to the concept of teaching children about emotion regulation, you can say something like,

Parents are the first and most important teachers in their children's lives. Children are dependent on their parents for everything at birth and slowly grow and learn to care for themselves. Until they are able to do things for themselves, they rely on their parents to meet all of their needs, including needs for love, affection, and emotional support. This is also true for learning how to behave and learning about emotions and how to deal with emotions in healthy ways. We want you to be really aware of your role as an emotion regulation model and coach because you are always teaching your child, whether you realize it or not!

Sensitively talk with parents about their own emotional experiences and reactions when parenting their child with challenging behaviors and strong emotions. It is likely that parents have strong emotions when parenting their child with ADHD, which can be really stressful. In fact, some people refer to parenting a child with attention and behavior problems as a *chronic stressor*. As much as the parent loves their child, the child may be hard to like or understand at times. As a result, parents may sometimes lose their cool in the face of frustrating child behavior. They might also worry about how the behavioral and social difficulties their child experiences now will impact the child in the long run. These emotions are normal for any parent to feel and particularly for parents of children with more challenging behaviors.

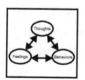

Here, you can refer back to the cognitive-behavioral therapy (CBT) (thoughts, feelings, and behaviors) triangle. Help parents to see that what they are thinking and feeling when their child expresses emotions or misbehaves affects how they react to the child. If parents put themselves in the role of teacher and model, they will need to manage their experience and use opportunities to coach their child when the child is having a difficult time.

> ### Goal 2: Help parents become more aware of and attentive to their children's emotions

Few parents view their child's negative emotions as a good thing. However, when the child is experiencing a negative emotion, this is actually an opportunity for connection and teaching ("a teachable moment"). Just as we asked parents to "catch the child being good" in Modules 4 and 5, in this module we ask the parent to tune their radar to pick up signs that the child is feeling a certain way. (See Handout 9.1: Child Emotion List for common emotions experienced by children with ADHD.) Sometimes it may be challenging to know exactly what their child is thinking and feeling. Depending on their age and emotional awareness, the child may not be able to articulate what they are feeling, but we can usually pick up (from their verbal or nonverbal behavior) that they are feeling *something*.

At these times, it is important for parents to practice empathy: putting themselves in their child's shoes and seeing the situation from their perspective. This can be incredibly challenging for some parents who are instead focused on the child's completion of activities or an expected behavior. Parents may quickly see something as not a big deal and dismiss their child's feelings. Other parents are more naturally attuned to how their child is feeling. Yet other parents may take on their child's feelings and feel responsible for changing them.

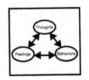

You can bring in the idea of the CBT triangle for both the parent and child in a situation (as the child experiences thoughts, feelings, sensations, and action urges, so does the parent; see Ehrenreich-May, 2018). You can say something like,

Imagine that your child is building something with Lego and is becoming whiny and feeling frustrated. You start to wonder why he just can't sit and build without so much support like your older child did. You are expecting an outburst any minute. You just know the signs that he is about to blow up. You also begin to wonder how on earth your child is going to make it in school as the work gets more challenging if he cannot even build a simple Lego! You feel your muscles getting tense and are about to lose it. Let's write out your thoughts, feelings, and possible behaviors in this situation. [Draw two CBT triangles and write the child's experience and the parent's experience for the same situation.]

Now imagine that you focus on your child's feelings. Instead of getting angry and worried about his inability to handle frustration and how this will play out in his future [note the cognitive distortion such as fortune-telling, catastrophizing, or labeling], you say "I can understand that you

feel really frustrated because building can be tricky and because you may think you won't ever figure it out," and see how your child responds. How do you think he would feel in response to your statement? How does this compare to your thoughts, feelings, and behaviors in the previous scenario where you can feel yourself getting into a negative spiral?"

A "negative or downward spiral" refers to when a lack of positive reinforcement in the environment (such as invalidation) contributes to negative thoughts, feelings, and behaviors, and this creates a feedback cycle resulting in increasingly negative thoughts, feelings, and behaviors that fuel one another (Lewinsohn, Munoz, Youngren, & Zeiss, 1986). Showing empathy for the child's emotional experience will communicate to the child that having emotions is normal and OK. By acknowledging their children's emotions, parents are helping them to learn skills that will serve them well for a lifetime. You can ask:

Can you think of a time recently when your child was having an emotion and you connected with them during this time? What about your interaction helped you to feel connected?

> **Goal 3: Teach parents to (1) validate, (2) tolerate, and (3) label their children's emotions**

After parents increase awareness of their child's emotion and begin to view it as an opportunity to connect, the second step is to *validate* the child's feelings and to *label emotions* (use emotion descriptions) to help the child express their feelings through words (give the parent Handout 9.2: Emotion Coaching). Pausing to allow the child to have an emotional experience and listening with acceptance provides helpful support when the child is experiencing unpleasant emotions.

Validation

You can say something like,

After you notice that your child is feeling a strong emotion, the next step is to say something supportive by using a validation statement. Your words and actions let your child know that it is OK to have strong feelings and that you understand why they might be feeling this way. "You are very disappointed," "It's okay to feel angry," and "I can see why you'd feel jealous" are validating statements that show your child that you accept how they are feeling.

We all have a tendency to try to use reasoning or logic right away, which can be *invalidating*. You can say,

Imagine you're feeling very frustrated with a stressful situation at work. How does it feel when someone jumps in quickly and tells you what you should do in the situation? Now compare this to how it feels when someone simply shows that they are listening and that they understand what you are feeling by saying things like, "That sounds really hard," "I could see how that would be annoying," or "Wow, that is so frustrating." Which helps you more in the situation? In which scenario do you feel better understood and supported?

Generally, feeling heard and understood helps us to calm down and feel better much more so than someone trying to logically solve our problem (even if the other person only intends to be helpful). A validating response like this also helps to build a stronger relationship with the other person. Instead of trying to reason, a validating response shows the child that the parent understands them and that their perspective is OK with the parent. For example, instead of trying to use logic to explain why something is fair or not a big deal, a parent can *first* validate the child's anger or frustration when the child *perceives* something as unfair or a big deal.

In *Emotion-Focused Family Therapy* parents learn to think of their child's emotional experience as an elevator (Lafrance, Henderson & Mayman, 2020). When a child is experiencing a strong emotion, the elevator may be on the fifth or even tenth floor. However, our ability to access logic happens on the ground floor. Thus, children can greatly benefit from parents first focusing on the child's emotional experience with validation and empathy before they jump to reasoning or fixing.

Labeling a Child's Emotions (Emotion Descriptions)

When parents validate their child's experience, they are using the opportunity to label the emotion. It is helpful for parents to understand the value of labeling emotions and the variety of ways this can be done. Using words to understand and communicate emotions is a **very** important part of healthy emotion development. By labeling the emotion and why it makes sense the child is feeling this way (the trigger), parents are helping their child to make sense of their experience. In addition to providing validation when the child is upset, parents can use emotion descriptions throughout the day when opportunities arise (see Handouts 9.1 and 9.2). Parents can label their own emotions (in a developmentally appropriate way; e.g., "I am feeling frustrated by all of this traffic"), they can label their child's emotions during Special Time (commenting on pleasant emotions like feeling proud or happy during play as well as unpleasant emotions like frustration), and they can point out emotions in others and the cues they use to know how someone else is feeling (e.g., "that person is feeling disappointed and I can see they are looking down and frowning"). Talking about the emotions of characters in books and with people with whom the child is not interacting can be another helpful way to help kids engage with emotion identification when they are calm. Parents talking about their own emotions gives children an opportunity to see how the parent is flexible or stays calm when experiencing unpleasant feelings. Parents labeling emotions helps to reinforce the message that emotions can be uncomfortable, but are not dangerous and do not need to be avoided. You can ask something like,

Can you think of a time when you used or could have labeled your child's emotion (used an emotion description) or taught your child about emotions? What was the situation and what did you say? How did your child react?

> **Therapist Note**
>
> Steer parents toward an example that does not involve misbehavior if possible so that it is easier to see the usefulness of validation. Demonstrate how to validate the child's emotion given the example they describe.

It is necessary and healthy for children to be able to experience and **tolerate** a range of emotions. By labeling the child's emotion, the parent is showing the child that they are not judging the child's emotional experience and it is OK to have strong feelings. Words that label how we feel can be calming ("name it to tame it"). Though this may not be the outcome in-the-moment every time, by consistently tolerating the child's negative emotions, the parent is teaching them that all feelings are acceptable and that the child is a person who is worthy of love, compassion, and understanding.

An iceberg is often used to demonstrate the idea that the emotion we see expressed outward (the tip of the iceberg) is not the only emotion the person is experiencing. We often see emotions like anger or frustration while other feelings like fear, sadness, or guilt may be hidden beneath the surface. Some children with ADHD and significant anxiety may experience frequent guilt when their ADHD symptoms interfere with functioning. On the other hand, some parents of children with ADHD believe that their child experiences insufficient guilt. This can lead parents to try to induce guilt (or shaming) or be overly critical of their child's behavior, rather than focusing on skills deficits like trouble with perspective taking and delaying gratification.

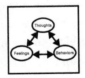

Therapist Note

For some families, it may be helpful to discuss the parents' concerns about their child's ability to take responsibility for their actions and to inhibit behaviors that have a negative impact on others. You can use this opportunity to provide education about these lagging skills and the impact of ADHD on social and emotional functioning. Help parents identify a supportive mindset (you can put these thoughts in the CBT triangle) so that their own critical or anxious thoughts about their child's behavior does not interfere with their validation of their child's emotions.

Another important benefit of tolerating children's emotions is that the parent sends the message that (1) the parent is someone the child can confide in now and as the child gets older, and (2) the child can feel safe and comfortable talking to the parent about any feelings they may have. This is an important message for children to receive from their parents because it influences how well they are later able to talk about their feelings, not only with the parent but also with other important people in their lives (e.g., friends, romantic partners, their own children).

Tolerating: What Not to Do

When discussing what tolerating looks like, it can be helpful to point out to parents what NOT to do (refer again to Handout 9.2: Emotion Coaching). You can say something like,

1. *DON'T distract the child from the feeling (don't give them something else to do so they temporarily forget about being upset): "You're OK, here's your favorite toy you can play with." Getting quiet immediately is not the goal.*

2. *DON'T minimize or deny the feeling: "I don't know why you are getting so upset about such a little thing." "It's no big deal, you are fine." Or, for example: Child says "I hate you" and Parent responds, "You don't mean that." Or: Child clearly seems scared of a loud toy and Parent says, "It's just a toy, you're not scared of a silly little toy." Denying feelings gives the message that certain feelings are not acceptable or that you don't accept your child when they have certain feelings.*

3. *DON'T negatively judge/criticize the child's feelings ("You're acting like a baby when you cry," "Why are you so emotional?") or suggest how the child SHOULD feel instead. For example: Child: "I don't want to go to the park!" Parent: "You should be happy you get to go to the park." Telling children how they should feel does not validate their true feelings. It's all right if your child is not expressing an emotion you would expect from them given a specific circumstance (e.g., sadness when a friend had to go home early, guilt when they did something wrong).*

4. *DON'T expect the child to be able to tell you exactly how they are feeling or give a logical explanation for why they feel a particular way.*

5. *DON'T connect your negative emotions to your child's behavior ("I feel very sad when you yell at me"). This might make more sense as they get older, when they are cognitively able to understand this (e.g., "I am very disappointed that you broke our trust and missed curfew"). For very young children, statements about how your child's behavior makes you feel won't change their behavior in the long-run AND it might negatively affect your relationship and their developing self-concept.*

Parents' Own Self-Regulation

As difficult as it is, it is essential that parents do their best to try to stay **calm** when their child is upset. Seeing your child upset can understandably be very upsetting to parents (especially when the child is acting out). It is also difficult to not swoop in and solve the problem to make the child's distress go away. However, it is very important for parents to stay calm and to model for the child that the parent can handle any emotion the child expresses. When parents stay calm, they can communicate the acceptance and confidence that will help their child with self-regulation. Parents can use the relaxation strategies learned in Module 5 to help them stay calm in these situations.

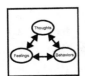

Of course, the parent will not always be able to stay perfectly calm. After all, they, too, are working on managing their emotions. When this happens, validate the parents' feelings and acknowledge that this is a process for them, too. They should not be too hard on themselves and should recognize their own improvements in this regard. (The thoughts-feelings-behaviors triangle can come in handy here.) When parents do lose their cool, it is helpful for them to discuss this with the child afterward (when everyone is calm) to process the fact that they were feeling upset, and that, although it is natural to feel that way under the circumstances, they should not have reacted in a harsh way.

Therapist Note

Some parents struggle a great deal with remaining calm when their child is upset. As difficult as it may be for the parent to engage in the self-care activities we have presented to this point, these self-care skills are essential to the parent's ability to remain calm. Gently revisit the self-care skills at this point using information about which skills seem to work best for this parent. Problem-solve ways that the parent can continue to incorporate these skills into their daily routine. Remind them how important taking care of themselves is for them to be in the best possible position to provide support to their child who is struggling. They need to "put on their own oxygen mask" before assisting their child!

Often, when children experience an unpleasant emotion, they act out in response to the emotion. The ultimate goal is to teach them to use emotion words (e.g., "I'm mad," "I'm sad," or "I'm disappointed") rather than engaging in aggressive or destructive behavior (e.g., hitting, slamming doors, shutting down) to express themselves, but this will take some time. For this reason, it is important for parents to learn to set limits while helping the child build problem-solving and self-regulation skills. Refer to Handout 9.3: Emotion Coaching and Misbehavior during this discussion. You can say something like,

It's important to remember that children with ADHD will not always calm down quickly and may not calm down at all. Sometimes your child will need a time out or other consequence if their strong emotions escalate to misbehavior. This is why it is important to remember that you should use consequences if needed.

Therapist Note

Make sure the parent understands when to use emotion coaching and when to ignore (or direct in another way). Sometimes parents feel unsure if they should be ignoring or providing emotion coaching. This can be tricky! In general, we suggest using emotion coaching to label the emotion once and to ignore thereafter. If the child displays a behavior that breaks a house rule or typically results in time out (e.g., throwing something, hitting), they can discuss the emotion later, after the negative consequence is given. Preparing parents ahead of time will make it easier for them to be clear on when to attend to their child's emotions and when other strategies are needed.

It is also likely that the child frequently will *not* be able to engage in problem-solving with their parent in-the-moment. Calming down and using problem-solving are very difficult skills for children with ADHD to use when they are in the situation and having strong emotions. In fact, many adults have not yet mastered these skills! It is important that the parents have reasonable expectations and think of this as a gradual learning process.

Praise Self-Regulation

It is important for parents to *praise any steps the child makes toward self-regulation*. That is, the parent should try to catch any attempts their child makes at self-regulation by giving labeled praises. For example

- "You are doing a great job calming down."
- "You had an awesome idea about how to fix this."
- "Thank you for using words to tell me how you're feeling."
- "I really liked how you listened to my idea about how to make things better."
- "I am so proud of your flexibility and thinking of a plan B."
- "Great job sticking with it even though it was frustrating."

Parents should avoid praising the child for *not* having a feeling; for example, they shouldn't say things like, "Great job *not* getting angry" or "I like how you are *not* frustrated." Rather, *encourage parents to praise for positive coping actions* like staying calm, being flexible, and persisting on a task.

Timing

Timing is another important consideration. Often, it is more useful to discuss an emotion and problem-solving or coping skills after the fact, at a time when the child is calm. In other words, it is helpful for parents to "strike while the iron is cold" when it comes to teaching. Provide an example like the following (choose a situation that is relevant for the child and family):

Yesterday you felt really angry when it was time to leave the park. I understand that you thought it was unfair because you hadn't had your turn on the swing. Today when we go to the park, you may have to leave before you've had a chance to do everything you want to. How can we help it to go better today?

It is important that these talks are very brief, being mindful of the child's attention span. It is OK that the child may not be able to stick with this conversation for very long. What's important is that parents are providing repeated learning opportunities for the child each time they have these conversations (i.e., taking advantage of teachable moments). No matter the outcome of each talk, parents are showing the child that the parent is capable and willing to talk to the child about any negative feelings or problems that come up in the child's life. By doing so, parents are building a strong connection with their child.

Role-Play

It can be very difficult for some parents to use the emotion coaching skills they learn in this module. Giving the parent a chance to practice in session can help them be more effective at home, *and* allowing parents to see how hard emotion coaching can be when things are calm (during role-play) can help them realize how little emotion coaching is probably happening naturally for the family. This role-play activity can be done with individual parents/families or in groups.

Ideas for Role-Plays

1. Ask the parent to describe positive emotions during a short play time.
2. Have the parent validate and tolerate unpleasant emotions during play (frustration with a toy or frustration when the parent does something they didn't like in the play).
3. Use a situation like homework, dinner, bedtime, or sibling conflict so the parent can practice validating and tolerating the child's unpleasant emotions in these situations. Ask the parent what the child does in the situation so you can act out the child's expression of emotion.

Have the parent label their own emotions and use an emotion description such as frustration in traffic, sadness about a change or loss (that would be appropriate for child to hear about), or worry about making a mistake or being late. During the role-play, praise the parent frequently, validate the emotions they may have when trying emotion coaching (such as feeling uneasy, helpless, or unsure), and make sure to let parents know when they do something invalidating or move into problem-solving or fixing.

At the end of each session, distribute the Parent Module Summary and reinforce the fact that the information discussed today will now be practiced at home. Home practice for this module includes

- Practicing emotion coaching skills (discussed later)
- Completing Worksheet 9.1: Looking at Connections: My Mood/Stress, Caregiving, Activities, and Thoughts
- Completing Worksheet 9.2: Special Time and Child Behavior Record Form

For Emotion Coaching Home Practice

Encourage parents to spend some time noticing which activities elicit strong emotions in their child (Handout 9.1). Examples might include doing homework, completing household chores (e.g., folding laundry), building a challenging Lego, doing an intricate craft, striking out in baseball, or losing at a game (e.g., Sorry, Jenga, Candy Land, Uno). Ask parents to join their children for these activities over the next week to practice the emotion coaching skills: awareness, validating, tolerating, describing, and setting limits when appropriate (Handout 9.2). During this practice, remind parents to use their own emotion regulation skills (e.g., relaxation) to stay calm and serve as an effective emotion regulation model and coach for the child. They can also take opportunities to practice emotion labeling when they themselves are experiencing an emotion that is appropriate to share with the child ("I'm feeling disappointed that my plans were cancelled") or to point out emotions for characters in books, shows, movies, or for other people. You can refer them to Handouts 9.1 and 9.2 for examples of emotions and how to respond.

Additional Resources

- *Raising An Emotionally Intelligent Child*, by Gottman (1998).
- *Meta-emotion: How Families Communicate Emotionally*, by Gottman, Katz, and Hooven (2013).

- *The Power of Validation*, by Hall and Cook (2011).
- *How to Talk So Kids Will Listen and Listen So Kids Will Talk*, by Faber and Mazlish (2012).
- *What to say to kids when nothing seems to work: A practical guide for parents and caregivers*, by Lafrance and Miller (2020).

CHAPTER 10

Module 10: Home Point Systems

(Recommended Length: 1 Session)

Materials Needed for the Module

Forms, parent summaries, worksheets, and handouts appear in Appendix A: Client Materials, located at the end of this therapist guide. You may photocopy this material for your clients, or you may download these items from the Treatments That Work web site at www.oxfordclinicalpsych.com/ADHDparenting. For an outline of this and all modules, go to Appendix B: Therapist Outlines.

Parent Materials

- Module 10 Parent Summary
- Worksheet 10.1: Weekly Home Point System
- Worksheet 10.2: Looking at Connections: My Mood/Stress, Caregiving, Activities, and Thoughts
- Worksheet 10.3: Special Time and Child Behavior Record Form
- Handout 10.1: Sample Weekly Home Point System

Assessment to Be Given at Every Session

- Form B: Top Problems

Home Practice Review from Module 9

In Module 9, parents were introduced to the concept of children's emotion development and learned how to serve as their child's emotion coach. Parents also learned how to decide when they should use emotion coaching versus behavioral consequences. You can use some of the following questions to facilitate the home practice review:

- *Did you label emotions for your child—either your child's, your own, or someone else's this week? Did you find opportunities to label positive emotions or label emotions during Special Time?*
- *What was your own emotional experience like when you tried to validate and tolerate your child's intense and unpleasant emotions? Did anything help (or interfere with) your ability to accept your child's emotions?*
- *For skills like problem-solving and perspective-taking, did you consider the importance of timing and wait to do these things when your child was calm?*
- *Did you have to manage any misbehavior in situations where you did emotion coaching? Do you have questions about how to handle misbehavior when your child is having strong emotions?*

Ask the parent to share successes and challenges in connecting with their child when they expressed an emotion. You can also ask the parent to share what their experience was like with validating and tolerating their child's unpleasant emotions. If it was difficult, ask them what coping strategies they used to help them accept their child's emotions when having strong emotions themselves. If parents report that self-care was helpful in keeping overall stress lower, make sure to celebrate this success with them. If stress interfered with their ability to do emotion coaching, spend some time thinking about what is feasible for self-care for the coming week.

Therapist Note

Make sure to adjust the home practice review based on what was assigned in the previous session. If topics haven't been covered yet, omit questions about that content from the home practice review. Also, if this home practice review does not include content that has been covered and given for home practice (e.g., if you are doing modules in a different order), make sure to expand the home practice review to include all assigned items.

Sometimes parents have tried everything to this point and their child is still struggling with compliance, routines, and perhaps other more serious behaviors. It is at this point that you can suggest a more intensive point or token system. The rationale for this type of system is that children with attention-deficit/hyperactivity disorder (ADHD) prefer frequent, immediate rewards over delayed rewards. For these children, praise is just not enough to change behavior. The overall goal of the home point/token system is to make the expected behaviors very explicit and to provide rewards or privileges contingent on an explicit set of behaviors, but with a more structured system of reinforcement. In a system such as this, children receive more frequent, tangible, or privileged rewards for their behavior. At the same time, they will lose points or tokens for misbehavior (such as breaking house rules; see Module 6). Privileges that were once provided noncontingently or arbitrarily (e.g., screen time, dessert, money) will now have to be earned. This type of system has the added benefit of allowing the parent (and therapist) to track progress over time in a more deliberate way.

In order for a system like this to work effectively, it must be implemented *consistently* by all caregivers—which can be very challenging for some families, for all of the reasons we have discussed throughout this program. Keeping the system simple and straightforward tends to work best, especially as parents are first learning the principles and skills. It may also be helpful to begin by focusing on one time of day (e.g., morning routine) to acclimate parents to the system and its principles, and then later expanding to other times of the day.

Specific goals for this module include

- **Goal 1:** Parents will come to understand that many children with ADHD need more frequent levels of reinforcement.
- **Goal 2:** Help parents identify specific and observable behaviors that will be targeted in the home point system, beginning with a discrete time of day.
- **Goal 3:** Help parents identify the currency (points, tokens, money) for their system.

- **Goal 4:** Help parents identify a reward menu consisting of both daily and weekly rewards.
- **Goal 5:** Address potential barriers to the success of the home point system.

Module 10 Content (Divided by Goals)

> *Goal 1: Parents will come to understand that many children with ADHD need more frequent levels of reinforcement*

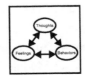

Many parents have a hard time accepting that they are being asked to provide the child with praise or rewards for behaviors they *should* be doing already. This expectation can be framed in terms of the thoughts-feelings-behaviors triangle. You can gently point out that the child is *not* doing the desired behavior (or refraining from the misbehavior) currently, for any of a number of reasons, which might include low motivation, difficulties with sustained attention, or pure defiance. This is why a more intensive and structured reward program may be needed to break down a desired behavior or set of behaviors and provide external motivators to encourage the behavior. Share Handout 10.1: Sample Weekly Home Point System to provide parents with an example of a home point system.

Some parents may view this approach as "bribery." If a parent says this, you can point out that we all operate on reward systems in our daily lives and in society. For example, we are rewarded for going to work with a paycheck; we get bonuses for a job very well done. Our children receive grades for their academic work. We often tell our children that they cannot have dessert unless they eat their vegetables. Or that they can go outside to play after they finish their homework. In other words, we have to work hard for the rewards we enjoy. This usually resonates with most parents. For parents who still seem skeptical, infusing elements of motivational interviewing (see introduction to this therapist guide and also Miller & Rollnick, 2012) can be helpful.

The behavior-rewards or behavior-consequences links are more formalized in a system like this and are therefore clearer, more organized, and more consistent. That is precisely what many children with

ADHD need to learn a new behavior. So this is not the same as bribery, where someone is manipulated to do an often illicit or inappropriate behavior. Instead, we are trying to teach the child how to complete daily tasks, which will help them get by in the world independently. The goal is for these frequent reinforcers to be temporary until the child is used to the routine and it eventually becomes automatic.

A side effect of a system like this is that it forces parents to *notice* when their child is doing what they are supposed to do (similar to Module 4), which has many positive trickle-down effects in terms of parent–child relationship, parents' own well-being, and family harmony.

> *Goal 2: Help parents identify specific and observable behaviors that will be targeted in the home point system, beginning with a discrete time of day*

Whichever behaviors or routines are causing the most impairment should be the initial target of the home point system. Most often these behaviors will include steps of a daily routine (e.g., the morning, homework, or bedtime routine; see Module 3) and/or the house rules established in Module 6. In addition, some parents allow children to earn points for completing chores like folding their own laundry or taking out the garbage. This has the added benefit of teaching responsibility and life skills.

As always, the target behaviors should be observable, clearly defined, and communicated to the child in a family meeting. The target behaviors should also be evaluated regularly, as they happen. Parents should always confirm that the behavior was completed before awarding points, rather than taking the child's word for it (e.g., with brushing teeth). Especially at the beginning, parents should be awarding lots of tokens/points to fully engage the child in the system and to get them excited about possible rewards. You can share Worksheet 10.1: Weekly Home Point System and say

We want you to begin with two behaviors that you wish to increase. Often, parents are tempted to work on several behaviors at once, but we want you to keep it simple at the beginning. You can add more behaviors after you get into a routine with the program. Starting with too complicated of a system can be confusing for both the child and parent, and it can be overwhelming to parents. In our experience, parents who begin with targeting too many behaviors at once have trouble using the system consistently and quickly give up. Others spend a lot of time creating an elaborate system with fancy currency or signs and seem to get lost in the details. By starting simple, you can master the system first before adding more target behaviors. Your child will also have an easier time understanding a simpler system.

Goal 3: Help parents identify the currency (points, tokens, money) for their system

The currency in a home point/token system is symbolic and only has value insofar as it can be exchanged for rewards or privileges. Older children may be most motivated by money itself, especially if they have a particular item in mind that they would like to buy or a place they would like to go. But, most of the time, tokens work well because they can be exchanged for a variety of different rewards.

 Fortunately, there are currently many mobile applications that can be used to keep track of points or tokens (as an example, see Rooster Money in the Apple Store). Multiple caregivers can log into these apps and reward or take points wherever they are (unlike a poster board they can only access at home). These apps also allow a parent to select their currency, notate why the child earned or lost points, and display their progress toward a goal that is visually depicted. Older children with their own tablet or mobile phone can also check their balance. Alternatively, parents can create a paper form in a checkbook format to show points added, deducted, and withdrawn.

Goal 4: Help parents identify a reward menu consisting of both daily and weekly rewards

Support the parent to work together with the child to generate a menu of various short- and long-term rewards. *Short-term rewards* are critically important because children with ADHD favor immediate versus delayed rewards. *Long-term rewards*, on the other hand, teach children to delay gratification and work toward longer term (delayed) goals. A *menu* is important because children with ADHD often lose interest in things easily, and a menu of rewards can ensure that they will remain motivated to work hard on the target behaviors toward their goals.

It will take some trial and error to determine how much various rewards should "cost" and how much the various behaviors are worth. These decisions should be made in consideration of the child's math/computational abilities. Working with increments of 10 is simple. For example, completing each step of the daily routine can be worth 10 points, breaking a house rule can cost 10 points, and more serious behaviors (e.g., aggression) may cost 50 points. Each time the child earns points, the parents should clearly and enthusiastically state why the child earned points ("You earned 10 points for brushing your teeth when you were told!" "You earned 10 points for getting started on your homework right away!"). Point removals should be stated in a firm but neutral tone ("You lost 10 points for not listening").

As noted, children can exchange these points for both short-term (i.e., daily) and longer term rewards. Examples of daily rewards are privileges that can be cashed in without much trouble: 1 minute of screen time (television, tablet, videogames, cell phone) per point; a special dessert; or time playing with a special toy. If the daily reward is to go out for ice cream or take a walk to the park, there may not be time to do this on a typical weeknight, and, as a result, the child will not be rewarded for meeting the goal. They may not work as hard to meet their goal the next day because they did not receive their daily reward.

Older children may simply like to receive the 10 cents, which they can save up for the longer term reward (i.e., the item they wish to purchase). Taking this approach, the money is the short-term reward and the item they wish to purchase by saving their money is the long-term reward. Of course, this approach has the added value of teaching older children how to manage money and save up for something they want.

In a home point system, children also work toward longer term goals that allow them to learn to delay gratification. Examples may include saving up for a toy or game, taking a special trip to the library or an arcade, or going to the mall with friends on the weekend. Parents can track the child's progress toward this longer term goal in a mobile app or a reward chart and should review the progress with the child on a regular basis to enhance motivation and offer praise and encouragement.

These reward menus should be refreshed as children develop new interests so that they do not satiate on these rewards, which will decrease motivation to work for them. Note that things like Special Time and reading should generally *not* be made contingent on behavior because these activities are critical for relationship and language development, respectively. Also, if children receive whatever they want from parents or other family members noncontingently, they will not be "hungry" for the rewards, and the reward system will not work. (Parents may need to use their assertiveness skills with overly indulgent family members! See Module 6.)

> **Goal 5: Address potential barriers to the success of the home point system**

Home point/token systems can take a lot of effort from parents. Be sure to tune into any thoughts or feelings that the parents express that may interfere with implementation of the system.

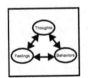 As noted previously, some parents are resistant to the idea that they should praise or reward expected behaviors that other children the same age do without extra incentives. Taking time to use the thoughts exercises from Module 4 can be very helpful here. The goal is to reframe this strategy as a temporary solution to motivate the child to learn to complete tasks and follow rules, which will ultimately help them to be successful and get by in life.

It is also helpful to return to the psychoeducation on the neurobiological and genetic causes of ADHD (refer to the introduction to this therapist guide. In other words, however annoying the behaviors may be (and we do want to acknowledge this), most children are *not* behaving this way on purpose. Rather, they need extra support and motivation to do things that are far easier for other children. Encouraging parents to acknowledge this is extremely important. But, at the same time, we want to encourage the parents to *foster independence* in their children because these are important life skills that will serve them well throughout adolescence and young adulthood.

 Other parents may buy into this type of program but simply not have the executive functioning ability or motivation to implement it consistently. After all, these programs can be a lot of work! Even more reason to keep this as simple as possible. Strategies taught in Module 3 can help remind the parent of supports and other ways to help them stick to the system. For example, setting alarms in the parent's calendar can help remind them to evaluate behaviors during a specific time of day ("Is the child up at 8:00?"). Having the home point system on an app that can be accessed easily at all times and can't be lost can also be helpful to enhance consistency.

Finally, in most cases it will take some time before the program begins to work. Given this, parents may not be rewarded for the effort they are putting in for a while. They will need extra encouragement and support to stick with it.

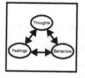

Therapist Note

As noted, in a home point/token system, it is critical that rewards not be provided unless they are earned. Make sure that parents agree that they have chosen things that will not be hard to give or withhold as needed. The tricky part here is that, prior to this system, many of the luxuries and privileges that were provided noncontingently will now need to be earned. Having to earn privileges and items that were previously noncontingent on behavior can result in a temporary increase in child misbehavior. It will be important to support parents through this transition period, using all of the parent cognitive behavioral therapy (CBT) skills taught to date (relaxation, constructive thinking).

Parent Goal Setting

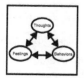

Before closing the session, ask parents to identify a specific target goal and reward for themselves. At this point in the program, the parents have learned about many CBT and parenting strategies but may have a hard time using them. Ask them to identify something that they could improve. Examples include going to bed by a certain time, doing daily Special Time, practicing relaxation, doing daily worry time or a daily success or gratitude list, or making lunches the night before school. Setting a specific and feasible behavioral goal for something that has been challenging, choosing a system to track progress, and designating a reward may be another way to help parents understand how the concepts discussed today can support their own behavior change.

> **Group Option:** Have parents work in the group to generate ideas using Worksheet 10.1: Weekly Home Point System. Have them begin by focusing on the hardest time of day and brainstorming the list of observable behaviors in the routine. They can use their worksheets to guide their family discussion at home this week, getting child input to enhance the child's sense of ownership. As a group, they might also brainstorm goals and rewards for themselves.

Home Practice

At the end of each session, distribute the Parent Module Summary and reinforce the fact that the information discussed today will now be practiced at home. Home practice for this module includes

- Setting up a home point system (discussed later)
- Completing Worksheet 10.2: Looking at Connections: My Mood/ Stress, Caregiving, Activities, and Thoughts
- Completing Worksheet 10.3: Special Time and Child Behavior Record Form

Setting Up a Home Point System

Have the parent work through the various components of their system with the child's other caregivers using Worksheet 10.1: Weekly Home Point System. Then have them begin with simply awarding points (liberally) for the first 3 days. On the fourth day, introduce the point losses. As noted in this module, it is best to start with one discrete period of the day to make this more manageable for parents and to allow for some refinement and success before applying this system to other times of day.

CHAPTER 11

Module 11: Review, Wrap Up, and Planning for the Future

(Recommended Length: 1 to 2 Sessions)

Materials Needed for the Module

Forms, parent summaries, worksheets, and handouts appear in Appendix A: Client Materials, located at the end of this therapist guide. You may photocopy this material for your clients, or you may download these items from the Treatments ThatWork web site at www.oxfordclinicalpsych.com/ADHDparenting. For an outline of this and all modules, go to Appendix B: Therapist Outlines.

Parent Materials

- Module 11 Parent Summary
- Worksheet 11.1: Effective Parenting Strategies
- Worksheet 11.2: Effective Self-Care Strategies

Assessment to Be Given at Every Session

- Form B: Top Problems

Home Practice Review from Module 10

In Module 10, parents learned how to establish a home point system. Parents learned to provide rewards or privileges contingent on an explicit set of behaviors, and they learned how to take points or tokens away for misbehavior. To review the home practice, you can ask

- *How is your home point system going? Did any issues come up that would be helpful to discuss?*
- Ask about the use of the response cost procedure: *For what behaviors did you take points away?*

It may be helpful to go through the point system developed by the parent in detail. Review their target behaviors, associated token/point values, and reward/response cost systems. Time should be taken to troubleshoot any problems that may have arisen and make any adjustments to the amounts being awarded or charged for various items on the list. If time allows, you can check in with parents about their other home practice (Special Time, relaxation, etc.).

Therapist Note

Make sure to adjust the home practice review based on what was assigned in the previous session. If topics haven't been covered yet, omit questions about that content from the home practice review. Also, if this home practice review does not include content that has been covered and given for home practice (e.g., if you are doing modules in a different order), make sure to expand the home practice review to include all relevant items.

Overall Module 11 Goals and Rationale

By this time, you have worked with the parent on many ideas for parenting and skills to improve their own mood and stress levels. Sometimes, without the ongoing support of a therapist, it can be difficult for parents to continue to use these skills consistently. The more consistently they incorporate skills and make them automatic, the more benefits they will see to their own and their child's well-being.

Another major goal of this session is to help parents feel prepared to handle future challenges that may arise. It is important to *anticipate* and catch problems *early*, so that parents can engage their tools before problems escalate.

Children are moving targets—once you figure them out, they enter a new developmental stage with new growth and challenges! Certain developmental transitions (i.e., to kindergarten, middle school, high school, and then eventually college) are particularly challenging for youth with attention-deficit/hyperactivity disorder (ADHD) as there may be new demands or expectations for increased independence. For example, the transition to kindergarten is a time when children are expected to sit for longer periods of time, regulate their behavior, follow the rules, and begin to complete work and other tasks more independently. The transition to middle school involves increased academic demands, coupled with organizational challenges like switching classes, having multiple teachers, getting longer term assignments, navigating new peer groups, and exposure to risk behaviors. College is another key transition period when a very high level of independence is required as the student is off on their own for the first time, left to manage their schedules, activities of daily life, and academics without the high level of parental support many have benefitted from previously.

In this module, the focus is on helping the parent to navigate these future challenges in the most effective way possible. ADHD is a *chronic* disorder so some form of treatment will likely be necessary over the long term, especially during these major developmental transitions. In this session the goal is to help parents to think about how they can apply the principles, skills, and strategies presented in this program to possible future issues they may encounter with their son or daughter. A primary goal is to ensure that parents have, by now, realized the value of self-care for themselves so they can create the most supportive and consistent environment for their children.

Specific goals for this module include

- **Goal 1:** Review the general principles of the ABC model and the thoughts-feelings-behaviors (cognitive-behavioral therapy [CBT]) triangle and reflect on how these models apply to the individual family.
- **Goal 2:** Help parents identify specific strategies that were most effective with their child.
- **Goal 3:** Help parents identify specific strategies that were most effective in maintaining their own health and wellness.

- **Goal 4:** Stress the importance of continued, ongoing monitoring of their own and their child's functioning so that parents know when to seek professional help.
- **Goal 5:** Instill hope and confidence that parents have the tools to help them through new developmental challenges.

> *Goal 1: Review the general principles of the ABC model and the thoughts-feelings-behaviors (CBT) triangle and reflect on how these models apply to the individual family*

ABCs of Child Behavior (Antecedent-Behavior-Consequence)

Begin by reminding parents that the more *consistently* they continue to incorporate skills learned in this program and make them automatic, the more benefits they will see in their own and their child's well-being. Moreover, children are constantly developing, and their needs and behaviors change. Encourage parents to think in terms of the ABC model in order to anticipate new challenges and prepare for their children's success. You may say something like

> *Children are a moving target—once you figure them out, they enter a new developmental stage with new growth and challenges! By using the models we have talked about here (ABC and thoughts-feelings-behaviors/CBT model) to think about and understand your child's behavior, you can approach these new challenges with skill and confidence.*

A critical antecedent to future problems is for parents to continue to use the tools that worked on a consistent basis (this will prevent or minimize problems). Sometimes, when things are going well, parents might slip back and not use the strategies as diligently as they did when they first learned them. However, encouraging parents to think of the behavioral parenting skills as a lifelong way of structuring their household and interactions with their family can help to make the skills more automatic.

Another example of an antecedent is to make sure appropriate educational supports are in place *prior to* a key transition (e.g., transition to elementary or middle school) so that the child is set up for success (rather than waiting to "see how it goes" without such supports in place). This latter approach essentially means waiting for the child to fail before doing what you know helps them.

If a *new problem behavior* begins, encourage the parents to think about the ABC's of child behavior: Antecedents, Behaviors, and Consequences. Where are things going wrong? Using clear expectations, rewards, and consequences immediately and consistently is key when focusing on a new problem behavior.

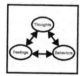

Parent Self-Care (Thoughts-Feelings-Behaviors/CBT Model)

Just like children, parents' lives are always changing, and we often face new challenges during adulthood. That is why it is important for parents to engage the CBT skills learned here on a regular basis to build up their "emotional armor."

We covered CBT skills by targeting

- *Thoughts*: Increasing positive/decreasing negative thoughts and changing thoughts
- *Behavior*: Pleasant activities, assertiveness, and social skills
- *Feelings*: Relaxation, mindfulness

If parents find themselves feeling especially stressed, short-tempered, out of control, or down, that is a signal to engage the CBT skills discussed in this program. Just as with their children, it is much easier to *prevent* a negative spiral by *prioritizing self-care* to enhance one's own well-being, parenting effectiveness, and overall family functioning.

> *Goal 2: Help parents identify specific strategies that were most effective with their child*

Worksheet 11.1: Effective Parenting Strategies, is a list of the parenting skills used in this program. Give this worksheet to the parents and ask them to reflect upon which parenting skills were the most helpful. Have them write these skills down (while their recollection is fresh) so that they are easily accessible.

Have parents reflect on what has been most helpful or salient to them in maintaining their own self-care using Worksheet 11.2: Effective Self-Care Strategies. What are the things parents need to continue to focus on in their own lives to maintain their own happiness and balance?

There may be skills that were especially effective for parents but that were *difficult to incorporate or maintain.* Troubleshoot with parents how to fit these things in. One common example is difficulty in finding time for their own pleasant activities (from Module 2). One solution could be to focus on the 1–2 activities that have the most profound impact on their mood. By putting this activity on their calendar (as we discussed in Module 3), it can increase parental commitment to doing it and can help them avoid scheduling over the activity. They can also bring in supports to watch the kids and adjust their schedules in minor ways to fit in some fun. For example, parents may get up a little earlier in order to take a walk, exercise for 30 minutes, or to enjoy their coffee and the newspaper before their kids get up. Or they may take a brief walk on their lunch break at work or during their child's soccer practice. Or they may plan to get into bed 30 minutes earlier so there is time to read a chapter of their book or meditate. Planning the activity with a friend can also increase accountability. Many apps exist for personal goals like increasing sleep and exercise that may also be helpful to keep parents on track over the long term.

The end goal here is to get parents to prioritize self-care and to make a lifelong commitment to maintaining this, for the good of themselves and their families.

Encourage parents to pay attention *on a daily basis* to their child's behavior and their own mood/stress level. The daily report card and/or home point system are important tools to monitor the child's behavior (Modules 8 and 10, respectively). Similarly, daily mood monitoring (Module 1) can help with "catching" oneself if one's mood starts to become more negative. It is much easier to catch problems early on than to pull oneself out of a deeper negative spiral. If parents have stopped using some of the tools that improved their stress/mood, it is time to start using them again! You might ask

- *What might come up in the future that may have a big impact on your child's behavior or functioning? How could the tools you learned in this program help with that?*
- *What might come up in the future that would have a big impact on your own mood/stress? How could the tools you learned in this program help with that?*
- *How will you know when it may be a good time to seek help for your child or yourself, before things get too bad?*

> **Goal 5: Instill hope and confidence that parents have the tools to help them through new developmental challenges**

You may ask, "How are you feeling about the future?"

We want to *instill confidence* in parents that they have the tools to help them through new challenges. The gains they have made so far in this program are due to the work they have done outside of the session. We want parents to *own* these changes, but at the same time let them know that it is important to get help and support when needed.

This program itself provided the parent with a great deal of emotional support. Work with parents to reflect on where they might get support as this program comes to an end. They may identify friends, family members, or professionals who can provide ongoing support. You may also suggest that they are now "getting back" at least an hour per week that they spent with you. How might they best spend this time in their own self-care?

> **Group Option:** Have group members discuss the following questions:
>
> - *What goals do you have for yourself and your child/family?*
> - *You have learned a lot and are ready to end the group. However, the ending of the group is a loss of regular support. How can you ensure that you have social support going forward? What types of group activities might you get involved in to replace this group?*

Parents have been part of a supportive group, and probably each member depends on the group and its regular meetings in some way. Parents should expect some sort of a letdown as the program ends and therefore *plan what they can do to deal with that.* For instance, they may want to attend carefully to their rate of *pleasant activities, particularly social activities.* Now is a good time for parents to consider how they will spend the time they would normally be in group, replacing this with a pleasant social activity.

Appendix A

Client Materials

Top Problems

(To be given in Session 1)

Date: _____

Name: _____

Top Problems—Parent

Please list the top three problems the parent is most concerned about. For each, rate how much of a problem it is, from 0 (not a problem) to 10 (a huge problem).

Top Problems	Severity Rating
1.	
2.	
3.	

Top Problems

(To be given in every session starting with Session 2)

Date: _____

Name: _____

Top Problems—Parent

Below are the top problems you told me about in our first meeting. For each, I want you to rate how much of a problem it still is, from 0 (not a problem) to 10 (a huge problem).

Problem	Severity Rating
1.	
2.	
3.	

Transactional Model of ADHD in Families and Foundations

Parents and their child with attention-deficit/hyperactivity disorder (ADHD) contribute to parent–child interactions and the parent–child relationship over time.

- Interactions between siblings and co-parents (e.g., conflict or support) also influence family functioning.
- School/community and cultural/social factors play an important role in expectations for child behavior, parenting norms, and the amount of support versus stress the child and family experience.

Beyond genetics and biology, these environmental factors play an important role in the degree of difficulty experienced by the child with ADHD at home, at school, and with peers. These factors can also contribute to the development of other problems over time (e.g., low self-esteem, depression, conduct problems). On the other hand, a supportive environment and positive parent–child relationship can protect the child with ADHD from negative outcomes and lead to more positive functioning.

Transactional Model of ADHD in Families

Cultural/Social Factors (e.g. support, stigma)

Parent Characteristics (e.g. ADHD Symptoms)

Child Characteristics (e.g. ADHD, disruptive behavior)

Parent-Child Relationship

Marital/Co-parenting Relationship

Sibling Relationship

School & Community Factors (e.g. communication, disadvantage)

Positive Processes (e.g. effective parenting, management of parent and child symptoms)

More Adaptive Outcomes

Negative Processes (e.g. ineffective parenting, unresolved stressors)

More Adverse Outcomes

Development of Child and Family Over Time

(Johnston & Chronis-Tuscano, 2014)

This program will focus on two things:

1. Helping you to be and feel effective in your role as a parent
2. Helping you to manage your stress and take care of yourself

The ABC model of child behavior includes three components:

- **Antecedents:** Situations/settings in which the child is more or less likely to misbehave
- **Behaviors:** Observable, well-defined behavior
- **Consequences:** Positive or negative consequences that happen right after a behavior and influence how likely the behavior is to occur again in the future

In this program, we will work on modifying the antecedents and consequences to encourage positive child behavior!

Things you would like to work on in this program (also referred to as "Top Problems"):

1.

2.

3.

ADHD in Families

Fill in 2–3 examples for your family under each factor listed here. Think about examples that impact your interactions with your child.

Child Characteristics

1. _____
2. _____
3. _____

Parent Characteristics

1. _____
2. _____
3. _____

Marital/Co-Parent Relationship

1. _____
2. _____
3. _____

Sibling(s) (if applicable)

1. _____
2. _____
3. _____

School/Community Factors

1. _____
2. _____
3. _____

Cultural Factors

1. _____
2. _____
3. _____

Looking at Connections: My Mood/Stress and How I Feel as a Caregiver

Mood/Stress Rating:

(1 = the worst I've ever felt to 10 = the best I've ever felt)

How I Feel as Caregiver Rating:

(1 = the worst day I've ever had as a caregiver to 10 = the best/ideal day as a caregiver)

Date	Mood/Stress Rating (1–10)	How I Feel as Caregiver Rating (1–10)

Special Time and Pleasant Activities

Special Time is very important to schedule with your child on a daily basis. During Special Time, you are giving your child your full attention without distractions, directions, or negative comments. Special Time can make the parent–child relationship more positive, and it sets the foundation for the rest of the skills we will work on in this program.

Special Time Dos and Don'ts:

- DO join your child for an activity they choose.
- DO give your child your full attention without distractions.
- DO describe what your child is doing, staying one step behind.
- DO praise your child for positive behaviors.
- DO ignore minor misbehavior (e.g., whining).
- DON'T direct your child, ask questions, or say anything negative or critical.
- DO end Special Time early if serious misbehavior occurs (e.g., hitting).

Scheduling **Pleasant Activities** without your child(ren) is a priority for parents, even though it may feel like you are too busy or that your kids are the main priority. By doing things that you enjoy on a regular basis, you will be in a better mood and feel more energized so that you can be your very best for your child and family (not to mention yourself!). This is *especially* important for parents when their child's behavior is challenging.

- What activities bring you the most joy?
- How can you fit these activities into your day-to-day routine?

Mood Monitoring: By checking in with yourself daily regarding your mood and stress level, you can

- Learn more about what activities bring you the most joy
- Notice when you are struggling and need support to bounce back

In this program, we will work on skills to improve your thoughts, feelings, and behaviors to help you feel and be your best!

Worksheet 2.1

Special Time Record Form

Date	What activity did your child lead?	What went well?	What was challenging?	How did you feel?

Pleasant Activities

Here, select 1–2 goals for pleasant activities in each category. Write when you will do these activities, and put it in your calendar.

- Relationships with Friends and Family
  - *Examples:* "Call my sister once a week," "Go to dinner with a friend"
    1. _____
    2. _____

  - When will I do this?

    _____

- Health and Wellness
  - *Examples*: "Get 7+ hours of sleep," "Go to yoga class," "Join a basketball team"
    1. _____
    2. _____

  - When will I do this?

    _____

- Spirituality
  - *Examples*: "Meditate for 15 minutes," "Go to church on Saturday"
    1. _____
    2. _____

  - When will I do this?

    _____

- Hobbies or Fun Activities
  - *Examples*: "Cook a favorite meal," "Crochet for X minutes," "Do a Woodworking project"
    1. _____
    2. _____

  - When will I do this?

    _____

- Education and Career
  - *Examples*: "Learn Spanish," "Go to a networking event," "Get my GED"
    1. _____
    2. _____

  - When will I do this?

    _____

Worksheet 2.3

Looking at Connections: My Mood/Stress, Caregiving, and Activities

Mood/Stress Rating:

(1 = the worst I've ever felt to 10 = the best I've ever felt)

How I Feel as Caregiver Rating:

(1 = the worst day I've ever had as a caregiver to 10 = the best/ideal day as a caregiver)

Activities that had an impact on my mood (more positive or more negative):

Examples: Talked to a friend, took a walk, had an argument, took a nap, watched TV

Date	Mood/Stress Rating (1–10)	How I Feel as Caregiver Rating (1–10)	Activities that had an impact on my mood (more positive or more negative)

Special Time Guidelines

During Special Time, you will give your child your full attention and follow your child's lead.

- Schedule a regular time to do 10 minutes of Special Time each day.
- Choose a time when your other children are otherwise occupied or a co-parent can help.
- Turn off cell phones and TV, and remove other distractions.
- Follow your child's lead during a play activity using the skills listed here.

Skill	Explanation	Examples
Description	When you describe your child's play and positive behavior, you are letting your child know that you are fully attending and interested in what s/he is doing. This helps keep your child in the lead. It might feel like you are a sports announcer!	"You are building a Lego tower with green Legos." "You are jumping so high." "You are painting your model car blue."
Praise	When you praise your child, you give your child positive feedback for their appropriate behavior. Try to be as specific as possible!	"I like how well you are focusing on ___ (task)." "I love having Special Time with you."
Avoid questions	Questions can be disruptive to your child's play. They can lead the conversation or lead the play. You may want to find out what the child is doing, but it is important to wait for your child to say what he or she would like to share.	
Avoid directions	If you tell your child what to do, it takes away their lead. Providing instruction is an important part of being a parent, but that is something you can do outside of Special Time.	

- If needed, ignore unwanted behavior (e.g., whining) until the behavior ends.
- End Special Time (for that day) for any aggressive or destructive behavior.

Module 3 Parent Summary

Maintaining a Consistent Schedule and Time Management

Children with attention-deficit/hyperactivity disorder (ADHD) function better when there is **consistent structure and routines** within the household.

It is important to set a schedule and routines around:

- Sleep/wake times
- Morning routine
- Mealtimes
- Homework time
- Bedtime routine

Because of their organizational difficulties, the parent and child can work together to break down complex routines into their component parts.

For some parents, maintaining structure and consistency is more challenging. Yet this is important and will help your child with ADHD function better. Consistent routines can also improve family harmony.

To stay organized:

- Use a schedule or calendar system
- Break down tasks into their smallest component steps
- Use a prioritized to-do list, focusing on what needs to be done now and what can wait
- Be kind to yourself and set reasonable expectations
- Be assertive about what you can and cannot do; don't be afraid to say "no"
- Remember to schedule your own pleasant activities!

By using these strategies, you will **model** time management skills for your child. These skills will help your child become more independent as they grow older.

If you think you may have ADHD yourself, consider getting evaluated by a psychologist.

Categorizing Tasks

Important & Urgent	NOT Important & Urgent
Ex: Comforting your child when they are hurt (do this right away).	*Ex: Going to the store to get milk (this task can be delegated or delayed).*

Important & NOT Urgent	NOT Important & NOT Urgent
Ex: Teaching your child how to ride a bike (can add this to the schedule).	*Ex: Making the bed (can be left undone).*

Worksheet 3.2

Looking at Connections: My Mood/Stress, Caregiving, and Activities

Mood/Stress Rating:

(1 = the worst I've ever felt to 10 = the best I've ever felt)

How I Feel as Caregiver Rating:

(1 = the worst day I've ever had as a caregiver to 10 = the best/ideal day as a caregiver)

Activities that had an impact on my mood (more positive or more negative):

Examples: Talked to a friend, took a walk, had an argument, took a nap, watched TV

Date	Mood/Stress Rating (1–10)	How I Feel as Caregiver Rating (1–10)	Activities that had an impact on my mood (more positive or more negative)

Worksheet 3.3

Special Time Record Form

Date	What activity did your child lead?	What went well?	What was challenging?	How did you feel?

Sample Routines

Morning Routine:

- Wake up at 6:45 AM
- Get dressed
- Make up bed
- Feed pet
- Eat breakfast at 7:00 AM
- Take vitamins and medication
- Brush and floss teeth
- Pack backpack with lunch and water bottle
- Bring instrument on Wednesdays
- Clear table and wipe down
- Get on the bus at 7:45 AM

Evening Routine:

- Pack backpack with agenda, books, etc.
- Pack instrument case on Tuesday evenings
- Pack sports bag on Wednesday evenings
- Take a bath or shower
- Put on pajamas
- Brush and floss teeth
- Read in bed for 15–20 minutes
- Lights off by 8:30 PM

Praise and Changing Your Thinking to Feel Better

Praise can be very motivating for children! Praising children when they are behaving and listening will increase appropriate child behavior. Praise should be **specific**, so children know exactly what parents liked about their behavior. Children can be praised for their effort and progress on a task as well as when they are successful.

There is a strong connection between how we **think** and how we **feel**. You can't always change the situation you are in (like when your child is not listening!), but you can change your thinking about the situation. Thoughts that lead to feeling very down or angry are called "**hot thoughts.**"

What are some "hot thoughts" you have about your child's behavior?

_____

_____

Thinking errors can make it hard to change our thoughts. Thinking errors are automatic, biased, and lead to negative feelings. After identifying thinking errors, we can **challenge** our thoughts and develop more positive and **helpful thoughts**. What is the evidence for and against each thought?

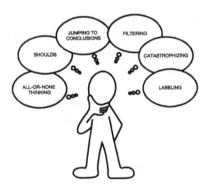

Strategies to **increase helpful thinking** and **decrease unhelpful thinking** can change the way we think about our situation as well. These include

- Rubber band technique (STOP the hot thought)
- Blow-up technique (think about the ridiculous extreme)
- Use cues (pair positive thoughts with daily activities like eating)
- Time projection (think forward to when stressor is no longer there)

What strategies will be most helpful to increase your positive thoughts?

_____

Catch Your Child Being Good

Give specific praise and attention for behaviors you want to grow:

"I like it when you. . . ."

"It's nice when you. . . ."

"That was great the way you. . . ."

"I am very proud of you when you. . . ."

Make sure to praise your child for following directions:

"I like it when you do as I ask."

"Thanks for doing what I asked."

"I really appreciate it when you listen right away."

"That's really helpful when you listen so quickly."

Remember: Always give your praise right after your child does something you want to grow!

Behaviors I will look for and praise:

_____

_____

_____

Worksheet 4.2

Practice Hot Thoughts and Thinking Errors

What happened? (Briefly describe the parenting situation)	What did you say to yourself (think) about yourself, your child, or the situation that led to the strong feelings?	What were the strong feelings?	Was there a thinking error? (Which one(s)?)	What are some new ways of thinking about this parenting situation that are more balanced and helpful?

Looking at Connections: My Mood/Stress, Caregiving, Activities, and Thoughts

Mood/Stress Rating:
(1 = the worst I've ever felt to 10 = the best I've ever felt)

How I Feel as Caregiver Rating:
(1 = the worst day I've ever had as a caregiver to 10 = the best/ideal day as a caregiver)

Activities that had an impact on my mood (more positive or more negative):
Examples: Talked to a friend, took a walk, had an argument, took a nap, watched TV

Thought Practice:
- Decreasing negative/unhelpful thoughts (interruption, worry time)
- Increasing positive/helpful thoughts (writing down helpful thoughts, pay attention to successes)

Thinking Errors: Did you catch a thinking error (labeling, filtering, all-or-none, shoulds)? Did you use a challenge question? What more balanced thought did you replace it with?

Date	Mood/Stress Rating (1–10)	How I Feel as Caregiver Rating (1–10)	Activities that had an impact on my mood (more positive or more negative)	Thought Practice (Y/N)? Strategy Used?	Caught a Thinking Error (Y/N)? Challenge Used?

Worksheet 4.4

Special Time and Child Behavior Record Form

Date	What activity did your child lead?	What went well? What was challenging?	What were your thoughts?	How did you feel?	Did you Attend/Praise: "Catch your child being good?"

Thinking Errors and Strategies for Increasing Helpful and Decreasing Unhelpful Thoughts

Thinking Error	How to Challenge
Shoulds. When you have rules about how you or other people SHOULD or MUST act, you feel angry or down when things don't happen that way. You can *wish* or *prefer* for yourself or someone else to be a certain way, but avoid "shoulding." (For example, "I should not make mistakes.")	*Can I accept myself and others as they are right now?* You can wish/prefer something to be the case but not demand it. Be kind if you (or others) are not currently performing up to your standards, or adjust your standards to be more realistic.
All-or-None. This occurs when you think in extremes like always, never, perfect, or terrible. The truth is rarely extreme. (For example, When your child has a tantrum, you think "She *always* does this.")	*Does this really happen always or never? Is this really awful?* Think in shades of gray.
Filtering. We filter out the OK/good things about a situation and are left only with the negative. (For example, You think "Today was the worst day" because your child got in trouble at school.)	*What are the positive parts? What went OK?* (Nothing is too small to count.)
Labeling. When we give labels to ourselves or someone else, we are ignoring a lot of information. (For example, You think "My child is selfish" instead of "My child has a hard time sharing sometimes.")	*Do I or someone else really fit the definition of this label (selfish, failure, etc.)?* Think of things as more time- limited (this time, sometimes) or changeable than a hard and fast label.

Interruption: Stop the negative/unhelpful thought by interrupting it. Example: When you have a thought like "I never do anything right" or "This will never get better," yell "Stop!!!" or say to yourself "I'm not going to think that right now."

Worry Time: If you feel you need to worry but many of your worry thoughts are negative and unhelpful, schedule worry time (less than 30 minutes each day) and save unhelpful worries for then. During worry time, make sure that all you do is worry.

Write Down Positive/Helpful Self-Talk (Thoughts): On index cards and/or in the notepad of your phone, write thoughts that are more positive and helpful about yourself, your family, and your parenting to increase positive self-talk. It is important that you believe the thoughts that you write. Review these thoughts several times a day.

Pay Attention to Successes: At the end of each day, write down three things that went well. What do you like about how you handled something? Some people practice gratitude by writing down three things each day that they are grateful for.

Ignoring Minor Misbehaviors and Relaxation

Ignoring:

- Removing attention decreases minor misbehaviors or annoying behaviors in children.
- To ignore, remove eye contact, do not say anything, and do not touch your child.
- Stay consistent—ignored behavior gets worse before it gets better!
- Return attention to your child once the ignored behavior stops.

Differential Attention:

- Provide your child with lots of positive attention for the "positive opposites" of problem behaviors.
- Be sure to use active ignoring and positive praise consistently—these work better together!

Relaxation:

Relaxation techniques can help to manage stress when in tense parenting situations. It is important to practice these techniques in calm situations first, and then use them in more tense situations. Techniques to practice include

- *Benson relaxation technique*: This approach involves focusing on the breath moving in and out while repeating a meditative word (such as one, peace, om).
- *Jacobson relaxation technique*: This approach involves tensing and relaxing different muscle groups in succession.
- *Mindfulness meditation*: In this approach, you notice your present moment experience without judgment. There are different ways to practice mindfulness but they share a focus on noticing what is happening (thoughts, feelings, sensations) with acceptance.

Worksheet 5.1

Special Time and Child Behavior Record Form

Date	What activity did your child lead?	'What went well? What was challenging?	What were your thoughts?	How did you feel?	Did you Attend/Praise: "Catch your child being good?"	Ignored chosen behavior (e.g., whining)?

Worksheet 5.2

Looking at Connections: My Mood/Stress, Caregiving, Activities, and Thoughts

Mood/Stress Rating:
(1 = the worst I've ever felt to 10 = the best I've ever felt)

How I Feel as Caregiver Rating:
(1 = the worst day I've ever had as a caregiver to 10 = the best/ideal day as a caregiver)

Activities that had an impact on my mood (more positive or more negative):

Examples: Talked to a friend, took a walk, had an argument, took a nap, watched TV

Thought Practice:
- Decreasing negative/unhelpful thoughts (interruption, worry time)
- Increasing positive/helpful thoughts (writing down helpful thoughts, pay attention to successes)
- Did you catch a thinking error (labeling, filtering, all-or-none, shoulds)? Did you use a challenge question? What more balanced thought did you replace it with?

Relaxation Practice: Do mindfulness meditation or use progressive muscle relaxation (PMR) or Benson breath clips from YouTube or apps.

Date	Mood/Stress Rating (1–10)	How I Feel as Caregiver Rating (1–10)	Activities that had an impact on my mood (more positive or more negative)	Thought Practice (Y/N)? Strategy Used?	Relaxation Practice (Y/N)? How did it go?

Progressive Muscle Relaxation (PMR)

Before you begin:

- Allow 15–20 minutes to practice this relaxation technique.[1]
- Find a quiet, comfortable place that is free from distractions.
- Get into a comfortable position. You can use a chair, a bed, or the floor.

The technique:

You will be tensing and relaxing different muscle groups in your body. The procedure is the same for each muscle group. First, you will choose the muscle group (e.g., your fist). Then you will tense it and squeeze the muscles in that part of your body for 5 seconds. You need to feel the tension, but do not tense your muscles too hard! Then let go of the tension and relax the muscles in that part of your body. While you do this, notice the difference between the tension and relaxation.

It is helpful to listen to an audio recording while you are doing the technique, preferably one with a slow, soothing voice. Taking deep breaths throughout the exercise will also increase the feeling of relaxation. If you notice your mind wandering, gently refocus your attention to the relaxation. There are now several apps available to walk you through PMR practice.

Muscle groups:

- Right hand (clench your fist)
- Left hand, then both hands together
- Biceps (bend elbow and tense upper arm)
- Forehead (raising eyebrows)
- Mouth (frown)
- Eyes (close and squeeze)
- Jaw (clench, biting down)
- Tongue (press against roof of mouth)
- Lips (make mouth into O shape)
- Neck and shoulders (raise shoulders up to ears)
- Chest (tighten by taking a deep breath and holding it)
- Stomach (hold deep breath and tense muscles)
- Back (arch but do not strain)
- Buttocks and thighs (pull buttocks together while pressing heels down)
- Calves and foot (curl toes downward)

Ending the relaxation technique:

Allow your awareness to come back to the room you are in. When you feel ready, open your eyes and stretch.

Adapted from Jacobson, 1929.

Mindfulness

What is mindfulness?

"Paying attention in a particular way; on purpose, in the present moment and nonjudgmentally" (Kabat-Zinn, 1994).

Why should you practice mindfulness?

Mindfulness can help you to notice your experience so that you may "pause" before you respond. Our automatic reactions in challenging situations are usually not our most skillful because we act from our judgments, feelings, and sensations without awareness. Mindfulness allows us to "pause" and recognize our experience without judgment, which enables us to *respond* rather than react.

How can you practice mindfulness?

You can practice mindfulness by observing the present moment with acceptance. During mindfulness practice you continually notice your experience (thoughts, feelings, sensations, and so on) without judgment.

1. *Notice your senses*: A common mindfulness practice is to notice 5 things you see, 4 things you can touch, 3 things you hear, 2 things you can smell, and 1 thing you can hear. You can also focus on one sense: look for things that are blue or a certain shape; only attend to one sense, like sound, and keep bringing awareness back to sound.

2. *Do an activity mindfully*: Common daily activities like walking, eating, drinking, showering, brushing your teeth, even washing dishes can be done with mindful awareness of the experience. During the activity notice sensations and give your full attention to the experience.

3. *Mindfulness meditation*: Focus on your breath going in and out. When you notice thinking, let thoughts go rather than follow the thought, push the thought away, or focus on the thought (which can intensify feelings). To let thoughts go, imagine the thought floating away like a leaf down the creek or a cloud across the sky.

Assertiveness, Effective Commands, and House Rules

Giving Effective Commands:

- *Make sure you mean it!* Do not give a command if it is not important enough to make sure that your child follows it.
- *Make it direct instead of a question.* Give the direction in a very clear, direct, and assertive way. Don't ask. Instead of telling them what NOT to do, tell them what TO do.
- *Make sure your child is paying attention to you.* Be sure that your child is looking at you when you give the direction. You will need to be in the same room as your child, too.
  - Reduce distractions (TV, video games) before giving the direction. Turn off or remove these distractions before giving the command.
- *Ask your child to repeat the command.* You don't need to do this every time, but you can ask your child to repeat the direction if you are not sure they understood or forgot what you said.
- *Give time for your child to complete the direction before giving another command.*

House Rules:

- House rules are for behaviors that you want your child to STOP doing, like hitting, cursing, or throwing things.
- When everyone is calm and relaxed, have a family meeting to brainstorm and decide on a few house rules.
- For the next week, when your child breaks a house rule, point it out to them. Example: "You broke a house rule. You hit. Next week, you will start having a consequence every time you hit."

Catch your child being good. Praise them for following house rules!

Communication Styles

Assertive: Confident, clear, shares own feelings and understands others

Passive: "Holds it in," doesn't share own feelings, needs acceptance

Aggressive: Attacking, ignores others feelings, needs power

Passive actions I do:

_____

_____

Thoughts that lead to passive actions:

_____

_____

Aggressive actions I do:

_____

_____

Thoughts that lead to aggressive actions:

_____

_____

Assertive actions I do:

_____

_____

Thoughts that lead to assertive actions:

_____

_____

Effective Commands

If a command follows the ideas we discussed, write Yes. If it doesn't, please write a more effective command.

1. Can you please pick up your clothes?

_____

2. Go clean up your room!

_____

3. (Yelled from another room) Start your homework!

_____

4. Pack up your backpack and set out your clothes for tomorrow. Then put on your pajamas, brush your teeth, and read for 15 minutes.

_____

5. Stop running!

_____

6. (While child is playing a video game) Do you want to come to the table? It's time for dinner and the food is getting cold.

_____

7. Play with your cars.

_____

Think about *when* you can use direct commands with your child. Write out several simple commands that you can use during this time (e.g., telling your child to put something in their backpack; throw something away in the trash).

1. _____

2. _____

3. _____

Worksheet 6.3

Looking at Connections: My Mood/Stress, Caregiving, Activities, and Thoughts

Mood/Stress Rating:
(1 = the worst I've ever felt to 10 = the best I've ever felt)

How I Feel as Caregiver Rating:
(1 = the worst day I've ever had as a caregiver to 10 = the best/ideal day as a caregiver)

Activities that had an impact on my mood (more positive or more negative):
Examples: Talked to a friend, took a walk, had an argument, took a nap, watched TV

Thought Practice:
- Decreasing negative/unhelpful thoughts (interruption, worry time)
- Increasing positive/helpful thoughts (writing down helpful thoughts, pay attention to successes)
- Did you catch a thinking error (labeling, filtering, all-or-none, shoulds)? Did you use a challenge question? What more balanced thought did you replace it with?

Relaxation Practice: Do mindfulness meditation or use Progressive Muscle Relaxation (PMR) or Benson breath clips from YouTube or apps.

Date	Mood/Stress Rating (1–10)	How I Feel as Caregiver Rating (1–10)	Activities that had an impact on my mood (more positive or more negative)	Thought Practice (Y/N): Strategy Used?	Relaxation Practice (Y/N)? How did it go?

Worksheet 6.4

Special Time and Child Behavior Record Form

Date	What activity did your child lead?	What went well? What was challenging?	What were your thoughts?	How did you feel?	Ignored chosen behavior(s) (e.g., whining): _____	Did you practice steps for giving good directions? How did it go?

Assertiveness

Assertiveness means someone letting others know what they need or want without being aggressive or passive.

Assertive communication includes:

• Speaking calmly and firmly • Being considerate of both people's needs and feelings	• Having a relaxed and open posture • Clearly defining boundaries (what is OK and not OK) • Asking for what you need	• Making good eye contact • Accepting compliments and criticisms

To increase assertive behavior:

- **Identify situations** that you may have difficulty handling assertively.
- **Identify thoughts** that make it harder to be assertive.
  - What are replacement thoughts that can help you be more assertive in that situation?
- **Assertive imagery** allows you to imagine and practice assertive responses.
  - After you visualize the situation once, change the details and practice again.
  - This will help when you are in the situation.

Home Practice:

Choose a situation where you can practice being assertive over the next week:

_____

_____

How can you respond assertively in that situation?

_____

_____

(After your practice) How did it go? How comfortable were you in being assertive, and how effective were you in asserting yourself?

_____

_____

Time Out and Privilege Removal

Using Time Out:

Time out from positive reinforcement is effective in reducing more serious misbehavior or house rule violation. Here are the steps:

GREEN

- After your child is given a clear direction, count backward from 5 to 1. Count out loud for the first several weeks, then silently after that.
- If your child listens, give them a labeled praise!

YELLOW

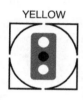

- If your child does not follow the direction, give them a warning and count backwards from 5 to 1 again.

RED

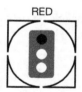

- If your child does not follow the direction after the warning, tell them that they have to go to the time out chair.
- Take your child quickly and safely to the chair.
- Tell the child to stay on the chair until you tell them they can get up.
- A brief time out is typically sufficient. The guideline is no more than 1 minute per year of the child's age.

RED

- After the time out is done, wait for 5 seconds of quiet.
- If your child was in time out for noncompliance:
  - Ask if your child is ready to follow the direction.
  - If they follow the direction, give a praise! Then give positive attention for appropriate behavior ("time-in").
  - If the child refuses, start time out again.

Additional Considerations:

- Time out for breaking a house rule does not require a warning—take your child straight to time out. When your child is done with time out, your child must agree that they will follow the rule for their time out to end. If your child does not agree, a new time out begins.
- Use a sturdy, adult-sized chair for time out. Place the chair in a place that is easy for you to watch but away from entertainment (e.g., TV). The ideal location is boring.
- Decide on a backup if your child gets off the time out chair (e.g., put them in their bedroom, remove a privilege, put them back on the chair).
- Do not argue or talk with your child while they are in time out.
- Contact your therapist with any problems or questions.

Time Out in Public:

Antecedents:

- Beforehand, review the 3–4 rules for this outing with your child(ren) and make sure they understand them.
- Tell your child what reward they will earn for following the rules.
- Explain that your child will go to time out if they break the rules.
  - Note: Think about *where* you can implement time out at the location (this should be a boring and safe space).
  - It is important to have some backup options (e.g., removing a privilege or ending the trip).
- To prevent misbehavior, get your child engaged in activities on the trip (e.g., looking for items at the grocery store or playing "I spy").

Consequences:

- Give specific praises for following rules throughout the trip.
- Follow through with time out if needed.
- Provide any promised reward if the child follows the rules.

Privilege Removal:

- For older children (age 9+ years) or for children who refuse to go to or stay in time out after trying techniques for at least a month, you can use delayed suspension of privileges (e.g., no television/electronics for the rest of the day).
- Parents need to make sure the privilege is one the parent can fully control (e.g., access to screens) and one that parents can follow through on (e.g., a parent can't take away the privilege of going outside if the parent can't physically stop the child).
- Avoid excessive/extreme privilege removal that you won't follow through on (e.g., losing electronics or no playdates for the next month).

Worksheet 7.1

Looking at Connections: My Mood/Stress, Caregiving, Activities, and Thoughts

Mood/Stress Rating:
(1 = the worst I've ever felt to 10 = the best I've ever felt)

How I Feel as Caregiver Rating:
(1 = the worst day I've ever had as a caregiver to 10 = the best/ideal day as a caregiver)

Activities that had an impact on my mood (more positive or more negative):
Examples: Talked to a friend, took a walk, had an argument, took a nap, watched TV

Thought Practice:
- Decreasing negative/unhelpful thoughts (interruption, worry time)
- Increasing positive/helpful thoughts (writing down helpful thoughts, pay attention to successes)
- Did you catch a thinking error (labeling, filtering, all-or-none, shoulds)? Did you use a challenge question? What more balanced thought did you replace it with?

Relaxation Practice: Do mindfulness meditation or use Progressive Muscle Relaxation (PMR) or Benson breath clips from YouTube or apps.

Date	Mood/Stress Rating (1–10)	How I Feel as Caregiver Rating (1–10)	Activities that had an impact on my mood (more positive or more negative)	Thought Practice (Y/N)? Strategy Used?	Relaxation Practice (Y/N)? How did it go?

Worksheet 7.2

Special Time and Child Behavior Record Form

Date	What activity did your child lead?	What went well? What was challenging?	What were your thoughts?	How did you feel?	Ignored chosen behavior(s) (e.g., whining)? _____	How many times did your child go to time out? How did it go?

Using My CBT Skills to Help Me with Time Out

Coping Skills to use **before** I need to give my child a time out:

1. *Assertiveness skills*: I can be assertive with other caregivers to let them know what I need to be successful with enforcing limits with my child this week. Do I need to delegate something to have the time to follow through? Do I need a change in the schedule so I can be home with my child to practice following directions (and time out if needed) without distractions? Do I need physical or emotional support to be able to follow through with the time out steps?

2. *Pleasant activities*: I can schedule pleasant activities to reduce my overall stress levels and improve my mood, which will help me to be assertive and calm.

3. *Relaxation skills*: I can schedule regular relaxation practice to improve my ability to use relaxation in challenging situations with my child, such as when I first begin to follow through with the time out consequence.

4. *Mindfulness*: I can practice mindfulness regularly throughout the day to improve my ability to use mindfulness in challenging situations with my child. I can choose a task each day to practice mindfulness (e.g., brushing teeth, walking, drinking tea).

5. *Helpful thinking/self-talk*: I can identify helpful thoughts and review them each morning to be able to use helpful self-talk in challenging situations with my child. For example, "My child needs to learn to deal with their anger without aggression. I can help them learn to do this by enforcing healthy limits." If I need to follow through with a time out in public, helpful thoughts include, "Others are often understanding," and "This will get easier as my child learns that I will follow through each time." I can put these self-talk statements on a notecard or in my mobile phone notes so I can also read them to myself during a time out.

Coping Skills to use **during/when** I need to give my child a time out:

1. *Assertiveness skills*: I can use assertiveness skills and act quickly. If there are many reminders or arguing or negotiating, there is more time for frustration to build for both me and my child.

2. *Relaxation skills*: I can use relaxation skills to feel better when doing the time out steps. For example, when my child is sad during time out, I will take calming breaths. Before I give the time out warning, I will quickly relax my muscles.

3. *Mindfulness*: I can use mindfulness to stay in the present moment without judgment of myself or my child. Mindfulness can help me to *respond rather than react* when I am stressed.

4. *Helpful thinking/self-talk*: I can use helpful self-talk to stay calm and follow through with time out. I can have a notecard ready and available with coping statements, such as: "One way I show my love for my child is calmly setting limits," and "I can help my child to learn that this behavior is not OK." It's OK to feel anxious, angry, or upset during the time out steps, and it is helpful to have reminders of things to say to myself in the moment to stay calm.

5. *Delayed response*: If I feel too upset, I can walk away until I can calmly follow through with the time out steps. I am an important model for my child, and my child learns a lot by watching me handle my strong emotions. It is better to take a brief break and return calmly to my child than to act with anger.

Working with the Schools

Establishing/Maintaining a Collaborative Working Relationship:

It is critical for parents and the school to have a collaborative working relationship to ensure the child's educational needs are met. In particular it is important for parents to

- Know the child's educational/legal rights under the Individuals with Disabilities Education Act (IDEA) and Section 504.
- Prepare for and participate in Individual Education Plan (IEP) and 504 meetings.
- Be familiar with evidence-based strategies that are helpful for children with attention-deficit/hyperactivity disorder (ADHD) in the school setting (for example, the daily report card [DRC]).
- Be assertive (not passive or aggressive) when communicating with the school.
- Be organized in keeping records of the child's report cards, disciplinary records, IEP/504 Plans, testing reports, evaluations, etc.
- Display good social skills in interactions with teachers and school personnel by expressing gratitude (thanking them) for their efforts, volunteering at school when possible, recognizing that they have the same goals (helping the child), and avoiding blame.

Daily Report Card:

The DRC allows for regular school–home communication, allows you to track behaviors and progress, and is an effective intervention when paired with short- and long-term rewards.

The steps in setting up a DRC are to:

- Identify the 2–4 most important behaviors that need to change.
- Define the behaviors in specific, observable terms that everyone has a shared understanding of.
- Pay attention to how often these behaviors are happening and set reasonable goals for a slight reduction. Goals can be adjusted as the child experiences success.
- Set up a reward system with daily and weekly rewards/privileges that are given consistently and only when the child earns them.
- Remember to focus on the child's successes and to problem-solve difficulties.
- Monitor and adjust the system as needed.

Daily Report Card

Child's Name: _____

Today's Date: _____

Goal Behavior	Period 1	Period 2	Period 3	Period 4	Period 5	Period 6	Period 7
1.	Yes No	Yes No	Yes No	Yes No	Yes No	Yes No	Yes No
2.	Yes No	Yes No	Yes No	Yes No	Yes No	Yes No	Yes No
3.	Yes No	Yes No	Yes No	Yes No	Yes No	Yes No	Yes No
4.	Yes No	Yes No	Yes No	Yes No	Yes No	Yes No	Yes No

Other Goal:

_____ Yes   No

Number of Yes's:_____   Percentage: (Number of Yes's/Total Responses) = _____

Number of No's: _____

Reward: _____

Additional Comments:

_____

_____

_____

Social Skills and Assertiveness

Social Skills:

When we are upset or stressed, it affects our social skills. It is easier to get angry or be more sensitive, when feeling ignored or rejected. We might criticize others or not join in conversations or make eye contact.

Certain social skills such as smiling or sharing what we have in common (for example, shared goals) lead to more positive responses from others. Using these social skills helps to set a positive tone when we interact with others and can improve interactions.

Assertiveness:

Working effectively with the school and advocating for a child's educational rights requires parents to be assertive. Assertiveness means letting others know what you feel and need without acting angry or prioritizing the needs of others.

Example: A child is not getting the accommodations for ADHD he needs in the classroom.

Passive	Assertive	Aggressive
You are the expert/ know more so I will follow whatever you say.	I am concerned about how my child's challenges are affecting him in the classroom. I want to make sure he is getting the support he needs to be successful.	You don't care about my child.

Describe a situation where you had (or typically have) difficulty being assertive:

_____

_____

What thought(s) do you have that make it harder to be assertive?

_____

_____

What is a replacement thought that will make it easier to be assertive?

_____

_____

How can you respond assertively in that situation?

_____

_____

Looking at Connections: My Mood/Stress, Caregiving, Activities, and Thoughts

Mood/Stress Rating:
(1 = the worst I've ever felt to 10 = the best I've ever felt)

How I Feel as Caregiver Rating:
(1 = the worst day I've ever had as a caregiver to 10 = the best/ideal day as a caregiver)

Activities that had an impact on my mood (more positive or more negative):
Examples: Talked to a friend, took a walk, had an argument, took a nap, watched TV

Thought Practice:
- Decreasing negative/unhelpful thoughts (interruption, worry time)
- Increasing positive/helpful thoughts (writing down helpful thoughts, pay attention to successes)
- Did you catch a thinking error (labeling, filtering, all-or-none, shoulds)? Did you use a challenge question? What more balanced thought did you replace it with?

Relaxation Practice: Do mindfulness meditation or use Progressive Muscle Relaxation (PMR) or Benson breath clips from YouTube or apps.

Date	Mood/Stress Rating (1–10)	How I Feel as Caregiver Rating (1–10)	Activities that had an impact on my mood (more positive or more negative)	Thought Practice (Y/N)? Strategy Used?	Relaxation Practice (Y/N)? How did it go?

Worksheet 8.4

Special Time and Child Behavior Record Form

Date	What activity did your child lead?	What went well? What was challenging?	What were your thoughts?	How did you feel?	Ignored chosen behavior(s) (e.g., whining)? _____	How many times did your child go to time out? How did it go?

Sample Daily Report Card

Child's Name: *Jameson*

Today's Date: *10/15/2020*

	Period 1	Period 2	Period 3	Period 4	Period 5	Period 6	Period 7
Goal Behavior	Math	Reading	Science	Social Studies	Writing	Special - P.E.	Special- Spanish
1. Stays in chair with 2 or fewer reminders	**(Yes)** No	Yes **(No)**	**(Yes)** No	**(Yes)** No	**(Yes)** No	**(Yes)** No	**(Yes)** No
2. Follows classroom rules with 2 or fewer violations	**(Yes)** No	**(Yes)** No	**(Yes)** No	**(Yes)** No	**(Yes)** No	**(Yes)** No	**(Yes)** No
3. Completes assignments with 80% accuracy	**(Yes)** No	Yes **(No)**	Yes **(No)**	**(Yes)** No	**(Yes)** No	Yes **(No)**	**(Yes)** No
4. Teases peers 2 or fewer times	**(Yes)** No	**(Yes)** No	**(Yes)** No	**(Yes)** No	**(Yes)** No	**(Yes)** No	**(Yes)** No

Other Goals:

1. Follows Lunch Rules: Yes   **(No)**

Number of Yes's: <u>24</u> Percentage: (Number of Yes's/Total Responses) = <u>24/29 = 83%</u>
Number of No's: <u>5</u>
Reward: <u>48 minutes of screen time (2 minutes per yes)</u>

Additional Comments:

<u>Jameson had issues with paying attention in class. During lunch, he got into an argument with another child but was able to calm down once they were separated.</u>

Emotion Coaching

Parents are their children's first and most important teachers for how to regulate their emotions.

The goal of emotion coaching is to convey to the child that we all experience emotions (both pleasant and unpleasant) and that even negative emotions are OK. They are actually normal! By sending this message, parents are providing a safe space for the child to express emotions.

Parents model for their children how to handle emotions, so it is important to use all of the skills taught in the program to manage your own emotions. By managing your own emotions, you are modeling for your child healthy emotion regulation.

Emotion Coaching:

When parents serve as their child's emotion coach, the child also learns emotion language so that acting out in response to emotions is not necessary to express how the child is feeling.

Emotion coaching consists of:

1. Being aware of your child's emotions and triggers.
2. Validating and tolerating your child's emotions.
3. Using emotion descriptions about how your child is feeling and why.
4. Setting limits while building problem solving and self-regulation skills.

Parents should avoid trying to distract the child from the feeling, minimizing the child's feelings, judging the child's feelings, or expecting the child to tell the parent exactly why the child is feeling a certain way.

Misbehavior When the Child Is Upset:

Sometimes when children are upset, they may act out by yelling at or hurting others. When they break a house rule, parents should follow through with whatever consequences were established in prior modules (e.g., time out, removal of a privilege). The situation and child's feelings can be discussed after the punishment has been delivered.

Looking at Connections: My Mood/Stress, Caregiving, Activities, and Thoughts

Mood/Stress Rating:
(1 = the worst I've ever felt to 10 = the best I've ever felt)

How I Feel as Caregiver Rating:
(1 = the worst day I've ever had as a caregiver to 10 = the best/ideal day as a caregiver)

Activities that had an impact on my mood (more positive or more negative):
Examples: Talked to a friend, took a walk, had an argument, took a nap, watched TV

Thought Practice:
- Decreasing negative/unhelpful thoughts (interruption, worry time)
- Increasing positive/helpful thoughts (writing down helpful thoughts, pay attention to successes)
- Did you catch a thinking error (labeling, filtering, all-or-none, shoulds)? Did you use a challenge question? What more balanced thought did you replace it with?

Relaxation Practice: Do mindfulness meditation or use Progressive Muscle Relaxation (PMR) or Benson breath clips from YouTube or apps.

Date	Mood/Stress Rating (1–10)	How I Feel as Caregiver Rating (1–10)	Activities that had an impact on my mood (more positive or more negative)	Thought Practice (Y/N): Strategy Used?	Relaxation Practice (Y/N)? How did it go?

Special Time and Child Behavior Record Form

Date	What activity did your child lead?	What went well? What was challenging?	What were your thoughts?	How did you feel?	Ignored chosen behavior(s) (e.g., whining)? _____	How many times did your child go to time out? How did it go?

Child Emotion List

- Afraid
- Annoyed
- Bored
- Calm
- Excited
- Frustrated
- Glad
- Impatient
- Lonely
- Mad
- Proud
- Sad

Other emotions my child experiences:

_____

_____

_____

How/When to Label Emotions:

When I validate my child's emotions: "You are feeling mad because your sister took that!" or "I can see why you would feel sad because you were really looking forward to that."

Describe my own feelings/model: "I'm feeling impatient because we've been waiting awhile!"

During Special Time: "You are feeling proud of your work on that building!"

For other people: "He looks sad because his shoulders are down and he is frowning."

Emotion Coaching

Step	What it is	Examples	Why it matters & things to remember
Become **AWARE** of your child's emotions	Start to think about situations that tend to upset your child or cause intense emotions. Notice these situations throughout the day and think of these as *opportunities to connect with your child* and *to teach them about emotions.*	Recognizing that your child becomes very angry when they have to clean up their toys and go to school. Noticing that your child is disappointed when they do not get to do what they want to do.	Triggers of your child's emotions may seem unimportant to you, but they are very important to your child. Being aware of your child's emotions and triggers allows you to be prepared to help your child. Use empathy to connect with your child at these times.
VALIDATE and TOLERATE your child's emotions	Try to be there for your child by taking their perspective. Show your child that you are really listening to them and that you are trying to understand how they are feeling. Be aware of your own thoughts. Use strategies to be patient and stay calm rather than solving the problem immediately for your child.	"It looks like you're feeling sad." "I can tell you're frustrated, everyone feels that way sometimes." "I would feel lonely too if that happened to me." "I can see that you're disappointed." **DO NOT distract your child from the feeling, minimize/deny the feeling, or criticize/judge the feeling.** **DO NOT problem-solve.**	It is important for people to experience a variety of emotions, both positive and negative. In order for this to happen, you will need to allow your child to experience emotions and express themselves, even if it is very upsetting to you. When you are able to tolerate your child's feelings, you are connecting with your child and showing you accept them.
Use **EMOTION DESCRIPTIONS**	Label your child's emotion and the trigger. Make this a statement.	"You're feeling frustrated because you're working on a hard puzzle." "You're feeling disappointed because your playdate got cancelled." "You're feeling jealous because I went on a field trip with your brother today."	Emotion descriptions help your child to learn how to talk about their feelings. You are giving your child an emotions vocabulary.

Remember to SET LIMITS when needed	Tune in to when your child's emotion expression escalates to misbehavior. Remember you may need to give a command and follow through with time out when this happens.	Your child hits sibling when angry (instead of calming down). Parent: "Time out for hitting." Your child throws a toy across the room out of frustration. Parent: "Time out for throwing things."	Have reasonable expectations for your child's ability to engage in problem solving. It requires a lot of practice!
Try to BUILD PROBLEM-SOLVING SKILLS	Encourage your child to identify the problem and generate ideas for fixing it.	(after time out) "What could you do to feel better? How can we fix this / make it better?" (after time out) "What can you do instead next time you are feeling frustrated?"	It is helpful to practice problem solving after the fact when everyone is calm. Keep these talks short!
Provide **LABELED PRAISE** as often as you can!	Give specific, labeled praises for the appropriate behaviors your child displays when they are having a strong emotion. Give praise for every small effort your child makes at handling their emotions.	"Thank you for telling me how you're feeling." "Good job staying calm." "I like how you keep trying even though you're feeling frustrated." "I'm so proud of the way you're calming down. You're using a nice calm voice." "I like it when you share your feelings with me."	Remember to praise specific behaviors (i.e., things you can see) that you would like to see more of, rather than praising not having feelings (e.g., not getting upset; not getting angry). You want to send the message that any feeling is OK, but give your attention to positive behaviors you would like to see more of when your child is coping with an emotion. Don't wait for your child to do things perfectly before offering praise. Praise motivates your child and reinforces any positive behaviors.

Emotion Coaching and Misbehavior

If your child is displaying a strong emotion and NOT misbehaving:

- Label the emotion and trigger ONCE. Stay calm and tolerate and align with your child quietly for a brief time (1–2 minutes).
  - Example: "You're feeling disappointed that your friend couldn't come over today." Remind yourself that this is a big deal to your child. Sit close to your child. Do not minimize the feelings or distract your child for a brief time.
- If your child starts to calm down, continue using emotion coaching for a brief time.
  - Example: Use thoughts that help you align with your child ("My child is having a hard time and needs my help"), provide physical support if your child likes that (such as sitting close or hugging) and continue to tolerate.
  - Then provide specific praise and convey confidence about next time.
- If at any point your child starts to misbehave during emotion coaching, follow the procedure outlined here.

If your child is displaying a strong emotion AND misbehaving:

- If it *can't* be ignored (e.g., breaking a house rule), then use the time out procedure or other consequence (e.g., removing a privilege).
- If it *can* be ignored, label the emotion and trigger ONCE. Stay calm and ignore minor misbehavior. Catch your child being good as soon as you can with a specific praise!
  - Example: "You're feeling mad that it's time to leave the pool today." Ignore stomping feet and give your child labeled praises for appropriate behavior (such as walking to the car, keeping hands to self, using calm voice).
- As soon as your child is calm, provide specific praise and convey confidence about next time.
  - Example: "I like how you told me about your feelings today. I bet the next time you feel disappointed when plans change, you'll do a great job staying calm and talking with me about your feelings."

Home Point Systems

Sometimes parents have tried everything to this point and their child is still struggling with compliance, routines, or more serious behaviors. This requires the use of a more intensive *point or token system*. The goal of the home point/token system is to make the expected behaviors very clear and to provide a more structured system of rewards/privileges contingent on specific behaviors.

Some key points:

- In order for a system like this to work, it must be implemented *consistently* and by all caregivers.
- Keeping the system *simple* and straightforward tends to work best. It can be helpful to begin by focusing on one time of day (e.g., morning routine) and then later expanding to other times of the day.
- Rewards or privileges cannot be given unless earned.
- Don't forget to *praise* appropriate behavior!

Things to consider:

- What are the *target behaviors*? Make sure they are clearly defined and easily observed. This can include house rules, chores, or steps of a daily routine.
- What is the *currency*? For example, will the child earn points, chips, money, an app?
- What are the short- and long-term *rewards* that will motivate the child?
- How will you *keep track* of the child's progress?
- How will you *involve* your child(ren) in setting up this system? A family meeting is a good place to brainstorm together.
- What tools can you use to *remember* to use the system consistently?

Weekly Home Point System

Reward 1 point each time your child meets the behavioral goal.					
Behavioral goals	Points earned				
	Mon	Tues	Weds	Thurs	Fri
Time/Routine:	Condition:				
1.					
2.					
3.					
Goal:	How it's measured:				
1.					
2.					
3.					
Daily total earned					
Rewards	Rewards received				
	Mon	Tues	Weds	Thurs	Fri
Daily					
Weekly (_____ points by _____)					

Worksheet 10.2

Looking at Connections: My Mood/Stress, Caregiving, Activities, and Thoughts

Mood/Stress Rating:
(1 = the worst I've ever felt to 10 = the best I've ever felt)

How I Feel as Caregiver Rating:
(1 = the worst day I've ever had as a caregiver to 10 = the best/ideal day as a caregiver)

Activities that had an impact on my mood (more positive or more negative):
Examples: Talked to a friend, took a walk, had an argument, took a nap, watched TV

Thought Practice:
• Decreasing negative/unhelpful thoughts (interruption, worry time)
• Increasing positive/helpful thoughts (writing down helpful thoughts, pay attention to successes)
• Did you catch a thinking error (labeling, filtering, all-or-none, shoulds)? Did you use a challenge question? What more balanced thought did you replace it with?

Relaxation Practice: Do mindfulness meditation or use Progressive Muscle Relaxation (PMR) or Benson breath clips from YouTube or apps.

Date	Mood/Stress Rating (1–10)	How I Feel as Caregiver Rating (1–10)	Activities that had an impact on my mood (more positive or more negative)	Thought Practice (Y/N)? Strategy Used?	Relaxation Practice (Y/N)? How did it go?

Worksheet 10.3

Special Time and Child Behavior Record Form

Date	What activity did your child lead?	What went well? What was challenging?	What were your thoughts?	How did you feel?	Ignored chosen behavior(s) (e.g., whining)? ___	How many times did your child go to time out? How did it go?

Sample Weekly Home Point System

Reward 1 point each time your child meets the behavioral goal.

Behavioral goals	Points earned				
	Mon	Tues	Weds	Thurs	Fri
Morning routine	Completes task without reminder.				
1. Brushes teeth by 7:00 AM		1		1	
2. Gets dressed by 7:10 AM	1			1	1
3. At table for breakfast by 7:15 AM					
Keeps hands and feet to self	One or fewer reminders.				
1. During dinner	1	1		1	
2. During homework	1	1			
3. During bedtime	1			1	
Daily total earned	4	3	0	4	1
Rewards	Rewards received				
	Mon	Tues	Weds	Thurs	Fri
Daily					
Outside play: 3 pts/1 hour	√	√			
9:30 bedtime: 2 pts					
TV/Electronics time: 2 pts/15 mins		√			
Weekly (15–20 points by Friday)					
Go to the movies					
Trip to the park					
Invite over a friend					

Review, Wrap Up, and Planning for the Future

The gains you have made so far in the program are due to the WORK you have done outside of the session!

Child Behavior:

- Think about new problem behaviors that come up using the ABCs of child behavior (antecedent-behavior-consequence).
- Using clear expectations, rewards, and consequences immediately and consistently is key when you focus on a new problem behavior.
- Continue to use the tools that worked on a consistent basis.

What might come up in the future that may have a big impact on your child's behavior or functioning?

Parent Self-Care:

- We have covered skills for changing feelings by changing:
  - *Thinking*: Increasing positive/decreasing negative thoughts and changing thoughts
  - *Behavior*: Pleasant activities, assertiveness, and social skills
  - *Physical Signs*: Relaxation, mindfulness
- Pay attention on a regular basis to your mood/stress level. Continuing to do your daily mood monitoring can help with "catching" yourself if your mood starts to become more negative. It is much easier to catch it early than to pull yourself out of a longer negative spiral.

What might come up in the future that would have a big impact on your mood/stress? How would the tools you learned help with that?

Effective Parenting Strategies

Note: The goal of this worksheet is to help you reflect on the skills that you found most effective with your child. Here is a list of skills that were covered in the program. In the table, write down the skills that you found most effective with your child.

Parenting Skills Covered in the Program:

- Special Time
- Structure and routines
- Praise and rewards
- Ignoring minor misbehavior/differential attention
- Effective commands and house rules
- Time out/removal of privileges
- Working with schools (e.g., daily report card, organizational skills)
- Emotion coaching
- Home point system

Skills That You Found Most Helpful:

Which skill(s) were the most helpful for your child?	How were they helpful?

Effective Self-Care Strategies

Note: The goal of this worksheet is to help you reflect on the skills that you found most effective for your self-care and happiness. Here is a list of skills that were covered in the program. In the table, write down some skills that you found most effective for your self-care.

Self-Care Skills Covered in the Program:

- Thoughts-feelings-behaviors (CBT) triangle
- Pleasant activities
- Time management
- Positive thinking
- Relaxation techniques
- Assertiveness training
- Social skills

Skills That You Found Most Effective:

What skill(s) were the most helpful?	How were they helpful?	How can I keep using these skills?

Therapist Outlines

To facilitate covering the material from this therapist guide in session, we have included a brief therapist outline for each module here in Appendix B. You can refer to these outlines in session as a kind of "cheat sheet" or "Cliffs Notes" until you become more familiarized with the program. In addition, you might find it helpful to return to the introduction for reference as needed throughout treatment.

If you would like to download these Therapist Outlines so that you can have a single page for each module in front of you, go to the Treatments That Work web site at www.oxfordclinicalpsych. com/ADHDparenting

Module 1: Psychoeducation and Theoretical Foundations

Therapist Outline

- Welcome parents and orient to the program
- Using Form A: Top Problems, ask parents about their top problems and severity ratings
- Provide an overview of the transactional model of ADHD and families
    - Give parents Worksheet 1.1: ADHD in Families
- Describe the first factor, Child Characteristics
    - Ask about child's temperament/personality and how it relates to child's behavior
- Describe the second factor, Parent Characteristics
    - Ask parents to share their characteristics that influence parent–child interactions
- Describe the third factor, Marital or Co-Parenting Relationship
    - Ask parents about the martial/co-parenting relationship, if applicable
- Describe the fourth factor, Sibling Relationship
    - Ask parents about their child's sibling relationship(s), if applicable
- Describe the fifth factor, School or Community factors
    - Ask parents about their child's school
- Describe the sixth factor, Culture
    - Discuss cultural context of parenting, child behavior, and mental health views
- Check in with parents about stressors affecting their family or parenting
- Introduce and draw the ABC model
- Discuss antecedents including examples of situations where child does best
- Discuss child behavior with a focus on specific, observable behaviors
- Discuss consequences
    - Ask parents for examples of positive/negative consequences they currently use
- Show parents Module 1 Parent Summary, and provide copy
- Explain mood monitoring and provide Worksheet 1.2: Looking at Connections: My Mood/Stress and How I Feel as a Caregiver
- Assign Home Practice:
    - Give Worksheet 1.2: Looking at Connections: My Mood/Stress and How I Feel as a Caregiver
    - Ask parents when and how they will do their mood monitoring

Module 2: Special Time and Pleasant Activities Scheduling

Therapist Outline

- Review home practice and Top Problems
- Explain the importance of daily Special Time and the short- and long-term benefits
- Give best/worst supervisor analogy
- Describe the main goal of Special Time, to follow the child's lead during an activity and distribute Handout 2.1: Special Time Guidelines
- Introduce the structure of Special Time, length (10 mins), and amount of talking
- Instruct parents to use <u>descriptions</u> during Special Time
- Explain <u>avoiding questions</u> during Special Time
- Instruct parents to <u>avoid giving directions</u> during Special Time
- Explain <u>avoiding criticism</u> during Special Time
- Discuss the importance of <u>praise</u> during Special Time
- Ask parents to recall what they will do and avoid during Special Time
- Discuss how Special Time can be added to the daily schedule
- Discuss appropriate activities for Special Time given child's age and interests
- Explain how to handle inappropriate behaviors during Special Time
- Role-play Special Time and emphasize parents being fully present and following child
- Introduce Worksheet 2.1: Special Time Record Form
- Introduce and draw the CBT (thoughts-feelings-behaviors) model
  - Define thoughts, feelings, and behavior in the CBT model
- Demonstrate how each part of CBT model is influenced by other parts
- Discuss the importance of parental self-care
- Give parents Worksheet 2.2: Pleasant Activities, and explain the mood-activity relationship
- Help parents choose 3–5 activities that are feasible, important, and enjoyable
  - Discuss how parents will plan to do the activities
- Give parents Worksheet 2.3: Looking at Connections: My Mood/Stress, Caregiving, and Activities, and ask them to track mood-influencing activities
- Distribute Module 2 Parent Summary, and assign home practice:
  - Give Worksheet 2.1: Special Time Record Form and Worksheet 2.3: Looking at Connections: My Mood/Stress, Caregiving, and Activities

Module 3: Maintaining a Consistent Schedule and Time Management

Therapist Outline

- Review home practice and Top Problems
- Discuss the importance of a consistent and predictable daily schedule to support children with ADHD
- Ask parents about how they currently manage routines and completing tasks
- List day-to-day tasks and activities with parents
- Work with parents to thoughtfully schedule daily activities
  - Discuss sleep, morning routines, meals, homework, bedtime, Special Time, and pleasant activities
- Discuss the steps of parent and child morning routines
- Give parents Handout 3.1: Sample Routines and review it with them
  - Help parents select one routine and break it down into the component parts
  - Discuss using prompts and praise for completing steps of the routine and a reward/reinforcer for completing the routine
- Introduce using a calendar system or review the parents current calendar system
- Give parents Worksheet 3.1: Categorizing Tasks, and discuss prioritizing tasks
  - Describe Eisenhower matrix and ask about current task/priority conflicts
- Discuss assertiveness and saying "no" when needed
  - Normalize the need to set boundaries with others to help manage time
- Discuss the need for flexibility and problem-solving within daily routines and schedules when there are disruptions like illness, travel, extra activities, or projects
- Distribute Module 3 Parent Summary, and assign home practice:
  - Implement changes to the daily schedule or routine
  - Practice using at least one of the time management techniques discussed such as use of a calendar system, a prioritized to-do list, delegating or not doing a task that is not a priority, or using assertiveness to say no to a request that is not a priority
  - Give Worksheet 3.2: Looking at Connections: My Mood/Stress, Caregiving, and Activities and Worksheet 3.3: Special Time Record Form

Module 4: Praise and Changing Your Thinking to Feel Better

Therapist Outline

- Review home practice and Top Problems
- Draw ABC model and explain how attention influences (reinforces) child behavior
  - Child <u>appropriate</u> behavior and caregiver <u>positive</u> attention should be paired
- Discuss "catching their child being good" to prevent misbehavior and specific praise
- Explain praising children for effort (as well as success) and progress along the way
  - Discuss praising "positive opposites"
- Give Worksheet 4.1: Catch Your Child Being Good
  - Have parents write specific behaviors to praise this week
- Draw the CBT model and discuss the connection between thoughts and feelings
- Introduce Ellis's ABCD model and go through an example using ABCD method
- Explain "hot thoughts" and go through challenging parenting situation example
- Give Handout 4.1: Thinking Errors and Strategies for Increasing Helpful and Decreasing Unhelpful Thoughts
  - Describe thinking errors with examples, focusing on most relevant errors
- Explain disputing the thinking error and generating a more balanced thought
- Distribute Worksheet 4.2: Practice Hot Thoughts and Thinking Errors to complete in session
- Discuss how parents can help children with thinking errors by modeling helpful self-talk and coaching flexible thinking when child is calm
- Discuss strategies to decrease unhelpful thoughts: thought interruption, rubber band technique, worry time, and blow-up technique
- Discuss strategies to increase helpful thoughts: writing down positive self-talk statements (priming), using cues, writing down successes daily, and time projection.
- Introduce mindfulness (presence without judgment) to respond rather than react
- Distribute Module 4 Parent Summary, and assign home practice:
  - Give Worksheet 4.3: Looking at Connections: My Mood/Stress, Caregiving, Activities, and Thoughts and Worksheet 4.4: Special Time and Child Behavior Record Form

Module 5: Planned Ignoring and Relaxation Skills

Therapist Outline

- Review home practice and Top Problems
- Review the ABC model and the rewarding nature of parent attention
- Introduce active (planned) ignoring and the benefits of using attention strategically
  - Discuss situations where child engages in mild inappropriate behaviors
- Explain differential attention as an effective way to influence child behavior, and encourage parents to praise "positive opposites" of behaviors that will be ignored
- Explain how to do active ignoring
  - Discuss expected reactions of child and normalize "extinction burst"
  - Emphasize the importance of consistency when ignoring
  - Help parents select two behaviors to ignore over the next week
  - Help parents problem-solve how they will handle the reactions of others when using active ignoring with their child
- Introduce how relaxation techniques benefit parents and that their ability to relax in more challenging situations will increase with regular practice
- Ask parents about past and/or current use of relaxation strategies
- Explain the Benson Procedure (focus on breath while repeating meditative word; see link in the module)
  - Practice the Benson Procedure in session for at least 5 minutes
- Distribute Handout 5.1: Progressive Muscle Relaxation (PMR), and instruct parents on using the technique at home
- Distribute Handout 5.2: Mindfulness, and explain how to practice mindfulness meditation (being present without judgment) in daily activities at home
- Distribute Module 5 Parent Summary, and assign home practice:
  - Give Worksheet 5.1: Special Time and Child Behavior Record Form and Worksheet 5.2: Looking at Connections: My Mood/Stress, Caregiving, Activities, and Thoughts
  - Remind parents of two specific minor child behaviors on which they plan to use active ignoring for this week (and praise positive opposites!)
  - Practice relaxation skills daily for 10–15 minutes

Module 6: Assertiveness, Effective Commands, and House Rules

Therapist Outline

- Review home practice and Top Problems
- Explain what assertiveness is (letting others know what you feel, need, or want) and why it is beneficial
- Draw and explain the communication continuum (passive-assertive-aggressive)
- Explain the goal of starting and staying assertive in challenging situations
- Provide examples of passive, aggressive, and assertive communication using a few different situations
  - Ask parents to describe their communication style
- Distribute Worksheet 6.1: Communication Styles
  - Ask parents to identify thoughts that make it harder to be assertive and help identify replacement thoughts
  - Describe and practice how to use assertive imagery to improve assertiveness
  - Help parents complete Handout 6.1: Assertiveness, and select a situation to practice assertiveness in their lives
- Explain how effective commands use assertive communication and make child compliance more likely (and show as antecedent in ABC model)
- Discuss guidelines for effective commands: necessary, stated directly, simple and one-step, have the child's attention, and consider the timing of the direction
- Distribute Worksheet 6.2: Effective Commands to complete in session
- Describe how to choose house rules (never-allowed behaviors, impulsive behaviors, behaviors a child needs to "stop")
- Discuss how to start house rules at home including discussing them at a calm time
- Distribute the Module 6 Parent Summary, and assign home practice:
  - Give Worksheet 6.3: Looking at Connections: My Mood/Stress, Caregiving, Activities, and Thoughts and Worksheet 6.4: Special Time and Child Behavior Record Form
  - Practice assertiveness imagery and using assertive thoughts and behavior
  - Identify several house rules, discuss them with the child, and post them

Therapist Outline

- Review home practice and Top Problems
- Draw the ABC model and review how changing antecedents (Special Time, routines, effective commands, house rules) and consequences (praise, active ignoring) have led to improvements for the family and child behavior
- Ask parents about current strategies for addressing misbehavior and rule breaking
- Introduce time out from positive reinforcement (TOR) as effective consequence
  - TOR is a predictable, consistent, and meaningful consequence so that misbehavior is not accidentally reinforced; helps with self-control
- Explain and model the TOR steps using the stoplight analogy with role-play
  - Explain how to take the child to the time out chair
  - Discuss the time out chair and placement
  - Discuss the procedures for when the child refuses to sit in time out
  - Discuss how to start using time out at home
- Explain how to use antecedents and TOR strategies in public settings
- Use the CBT model to identify thoughts, feelings, and actions that occur when parents are in challenging situations with child noncompliance or rule breaking
- Use Handout 7.1: *Using my CBT Skills to Help Me with Time Out* to develop a coping plan to help support parents' use of TOR
  - Incorporate assertiveness, relaxation, mindfulness, helpful thinking, and pleasant activities for parents as they establish TOR consequence at home
- Ask about and address concerns that remain around the use of TOR
- Distribute Module 7 Parent Summary, and assign home practice:
  - Give Worksheet 7.1: *Looking at Connections: My Mood/Stress, Caregiving, Activities, and Thoughts* and Worksheet 7.2: *Special Time and Child Behavior Record Form*
  - Show parents there is a new column to track if child goes to time out
  - Emphasize the importance of continuing daily Special Time when TOR begins

Module 8: Working Effectively with the Schools

Therapist Outline

- Review home practice and Top Problems
- Discuss the importance of establishing and maintaining a collaborative working relationship with the school
- Discuss accommodations the child may be eligible for and help parents to understand the child's educational rights
  - Give template (see link in the module) to ask for child's need for a 504 Plan or Individual Education Plan (IEP) to be evaluated
- Provide an overview of evidence-based approaches to managing classroom behavior
  - Describe use of behavioral strategies by teachers (influencing antecedents and consequences) and explain the range of possible accommodations
- Give Handout 8.1: Sample Daily Report Card, as well as Worksheet 8.1: Daily Report Card, to parents and help parents set up a daily report card (DRC)
- Describe how parents' ability to be skillful in social situations may be impacted when parents are upset and how they can use social skills when interacting with school
- Discuss how assertive communication can be used in school communication
  - Draw passive-assertive-aggressive communication continuum and give examples of school–parent communications for each style
- Hand out Worksheet 8.2: Social Skills and Assertiveness, and complete the assertiveness section as in-session activity
- Discuss strategies to prepare for and actively participate in all meetings related to their child's academic plan
  - These strategies can include organizing materials, identifying others who can advocate in meetings, knowing their rights, and plans for coping and self-care
- Distribute Module 8 Parent Summary, and assign home practice:
  - Take action steps toward identified school-related goals
  - Give Worksheet 8.3: Looking at Connections: My Mood/Stress, Caregiving, Activities, and Thoughts and Worksheet 8.4: Special Time and Child Behavior Record Form

Module 9: Emotion Coaching

Therapist Outline

- Review home practice and Top Problems
- Discuss the important role parents play as teachers in emotion regulation
- Discuss the challenges for parent emotion regulation in difficult parenting situations
  - Draw CBT (thoughts-feelings-behavior) model to show parents' experience when their child is having strong emotions
  - Add a second CBT triangle to show child's thoughts, feelings, and behaviors when very upset
- Share the important idea that emotions are a time to connect and support the child
- Give parents Handout 9.1: Child Emotion List and Handout 9.2: Emotion Coaching, and explain how to validate their children's emotions (accepting child's emotions without judgment)
- Explain the importance of emotion labeling and help parents identify recent situation where they used (or could have used) emotion labeling (see Handout 9.1)
- Discuss the importance of children being able to tolerate a range of emotions and that parents use of emotion coaching skills will help their child to do this
- Explain what tolerating does not look like (on Handout 9.2: Emotion Coaching)
  - Don't distract, minimize, deny, judge, expect child to be logical, or have child be responsible for parents' emotions
- Discuss the importance of parents' own self-regulation (CBT skills learned can help!)
- Give parents Handout 9.3: Emotion Coaching and Misbehavior, and discuss how to decide when to use emotion coaching and when limit setting is needed
- Encourage parents to praise efforts to cope with strong emotions and give examples
- Explain the importance of timing when teaching coping skills or helping child to problem-solve (prior to or after intense emotions, "strike while the iron is cold")
- Role-play emotion coaching skills with parents
- Distribute Module 9 Parent Summary, any Module 9 handouts that have not been distributed yet, and assign home practice:
  - Give Worksheet 9.1: Looking at Connections: My Mood/Stress, Caregiving, Activities, and Thoughts and Worksheet 9.2: Special Time and Child Behavior Form
  - Find opportunities for emotion coaching

Module 10: Home Point Systems

Therapist Outline

- Review home practice and Top Problems
- Provide rationale for the use of a more frequent, intensive, and structured reward system for some behavioral goals
- Discuss the benefits of a reward system in which behaviors are more clearly tied to privileges
  - Share Handout 10.1: Sample Weekly Home Point System to show example
- Help parents identify two specific, observable behaviors to target increasing with the home point system
  - Give parents Worksheet 10.1: Weekly Home Point System
- Help parents identify a currency for their home points system
- Help parents identify a reward menu with short-term and long-term rewards
- Address any barriers to the home point system
- Discuss the importance of not providing a reward unless it is earned
- Ask parents to identify a specific target goal and reward for themselves
- Distribute Module 10 Parent Summary, and assign home practice:
  - Give Worksheet 10.2: Looking at Connections: My Mood/Stress, Caregiving, Activities, and Thoughts and Worksheet 10.3: Special Time and Child Behavior Record Form
  - Set up a home point system

Module 11: Review, Wrap Up, and Planning for the Future

Therapist Outline

- Review home practice and Top Problems
- Convey confidence that the parents have learned skills that will help them throughout their child's developmental stages when used consistently and proactively (when possible)
- Review the ABC model and give examples of how this can be used for future transitions and problem behaviors
- Review the thoughts-feelings-behavior triangle (CBT model) and how it can be used on an ongoing basis to improve mood, decrease stress, and prevent a negative spiral
- Provide Worksheet 11.1: Effective Parenting Strategies, and have parents reflect on which skills are the most helpful for their child and family
- Give Worksheet 11.2: Effective Self-Care Strategies, and ask parents to think about the self-care strategies that are most effective for them
    - Discuss skills that were effective but difficult to implement or maintain to help parents problem-solve and encourage ongoing use of skills
- Discuss the importance of continued monitoring of child behavior and their mood/stress level to catch things early and to determine if more support is needed
- Discuss sources of support for parents and family as the program comes to an end
- Hand out Module 11 Parent Summary

References

Barkley, R. A. (2013). *Defiant children: A clinician's manual for assessment and parent training* (3rd ed.). New York: Guilford.

Baumrind, D. (1966). Effects of authoritative parental control on child behavior. *Child Development, 37*(4), 887–907. doi:10.2307/1126611

Beck, A. T. (Ed.). (1979). *Cognitive therapy of depression*. New York: Guilford.

Beck, J. S. (2011). *Cognitive therapy, second edition: Basics and beyond* (2nd ed.). New York: Guilford.

Benson, H., Beary, J. F., & Carol, M. P. (1974). The relaxation response. *Psychiatry: Interpersonal and Biological Processes, 37*(1), 37–46. doi:10.1080/00332747.1974.11023785

Bögels, S., & Restifo, K. (2014). *Mindful parenting: A guide for mental health practitioners*. Berlin: Springer Science & Business Media.

Boyce, T. W. (2019). *The orchid and the dandelion: Why some children struggle and how all can thrive*. New York: Knopf.

Castellanos, F. X., & Tannock, R. (2002). Neuroscience of attention-deficit/hyperactivity disorder: The search for endophenotypes. *Nature Reviews Neuroscience, 3*(8), 617–628. doi:10.1038/nrn896

Chronis, A. M., Lahey, B. B., Pelham Jr, W. E., Kipp, H. L., Baumann, B. L., & Lee, S. S. (2003). Psychopathology and substance abuse in parents of young children with attention-deficit/hyperactivity disorder. *Journal of the American Academy of Child & Adolescent Psychiatry, 42*(12), 1424–1432. doi:10.1097/00004583-200312000-00009

Chronis, A. M., Lahey, B. B., Pelham Jr, W. E., Williams, S. H., Baumann, B. L., Kipp, H., . . . Rathouz, P. J. (2007). Maternal depression and early positive parenting predict future conduct problems in young children with attention-deficit/hyperactivity disorder. *Developmental Psychology, 43*(1), 70–82. doi:10.1037/0012-1649.43.1.70

Chronis-Tuscano, A., Clarke, T. L., O'Brien, K. A., Raggi, V. L., Diaz, Y., Mintz, A. D., . . . Seeley, J. (2013). Development and preliminary evaluation of an integrated treatment targeting parenting and depressive symptoms in mothers of children with attention-deficit/hyperactivity disorder. *Journal of Consulting and Clinical Psychology, 81*(5), 918–925. doi:10.1037%2Fa0032112

Chronis-Tuscano, A., Lewis-Morrarty, E., Woods, K. E., O'Brien, K. A., Mazursky-Horowitz, H., & Thomas, S. R. (2016). Parent–child interaction therapy with emotion coaching for preschoolers with attention-deficit/hyperactivity disorder. *Cognitive and Behavioral Practice, 23*(1), 62–78. doi:10.1016/j.cbpra.2014.11.001

Chronis-Tuscano, A., Raggi, V. L., Clarke, T. L., Rooney, M. E., Diaz, Y., & Pian, J. (2008). Associations between maternal attention-deficit/hyperactivity disorder symptoms and parenting. *Journal of Abnormal Child Psychology, 36*(8), 1237–1250. doi:10.1007/s10802-008-9246-4

Duncan, L. G. (2007). *Assessment of mindful parenting among families of early adolescents: Development and validation of the Interpersonal Mindfulness in Parenting Scale* (Doctoral dissertation). Retrieved from https://etda.libraries.psu.edu/catalog/7740

DuPaul, G. J., Chronis-Tuscano, A., Danielson, M. L., & Visser, S. N. (2019). Predictors of receipt of school services in a national sample of youth with ADHD. *Journal of Attention Disorders, 23*(11), 1303–1319. doi:10.1177/1087054718816169

Ehrenreich-May, J., Kennedy, S. M., Sherman, J. A., Bilek, E. L., Buzzella, B. A., Bennett, S. M., & Barlow, D. H. (2018). *Unified protocols for transdiagnostic treatment of emotional disorders in children and adolescents: Therapist guide.* Oxford: Oxford University Press.

Ellis, A. E., & Grieger, R. M. (1986). *Handbook of rational-emotive therapy, Vol. 2.* New York: Springer.

Evans, S. W., Owens, J. S., Wymbs, B. T., & Ray, A. R. (2018). Evidence-based psychosocial treatments for children and adolescents with attention deficit/hyperactivity disorder. *Journal of Clinical Child & Adolescent Psychology, 47*(2), 157–198. doi:10.1080/15374416.2017.1390757

Eyberg, S., & Funderburk, B. (2011). *Parent-child interaction therapy protocol.* Gainesville: PCIT International.

Faber, A., & Mazlish, E. (2012). *How to talk so kids will listen & listen so kids will talk.* New York: Simon and Schuster.

Fabiano, G. A. (2016). *Interventions for disruptive behaviors: Reducing problems and building skills.* New York: Guilford.

Faraone, S. V., Perlis, R. H., Doyle, A. E., Smoller, J. W., Goralnick, J. J., Holmgren, M. A., & Sklar, P. (2005). Molecular genetics of attention-deficit/hyperactivity disorder. *Biological Psychiatry, 57*(11), 1313–1323. doi:10.1016/j.biopsych.2004.11.024

Franke, B., Faraone, S. V., Asherson, P., Buitelaar, J., Bau, C. H. D., Ramos-Quiroga, J. A., . . . Reif, A.; International Multicentre persistent ADHD Collaboration. (2012). The genetics of attention deficit/hyperactivity disorder in adults, a review. *Molecular Psychiatry, 17*(10), 960–987. doi:10.1038/mp.2011.138

Gawrilow, C., Stadler, G., Langguth, N., Naumann, A., & Boeck, A. (2016). Physical activity, affect, and cognition in children with symptoms of ADHD. *Journal of Attention Disorders*, *20*(2), 151–162. doi:10.1177/ 1087054713493318

Gottman, J. (1998). *Raising an emotionally intelligent child: The heart of parenting*. New York: Simon & Schuster.

Gottman, J. M., Katz, L. F., & Hooven, C. (2013). *Meta-emotion: How families communicate emotionally*. Mahwah, NJ: Routledge.

Graziano, P. A., Garcia, A. M., & Landis, T. D. (2018). To fidget or not to fidget, that is the question: A systematic classroom evaluation of fidget spinners among young children with ADHD. *Journal of Attention Disorders*, *24*(1), 163–171. doi:10.1177/1087054718770009

Griest, D. L., Forehand, R., Rogers, T., Breiner, J., Furey, W., & Williams, C. A. (1982). Effects of parent enhancement therapy on the treatment outcome and generalization of a parent training program. *Behavior Research & Therapy*, *20*(5), 429–436. doi:10.1016/ 0005-7967(82)90064-x

Hall, K. D., & Cook, M. (2011). *The Power of Validation*. Oakland, CA: New Harbinger.

Harold, G. T., Leve, L. D., Barrett, D., Elam, K., Neiderhiser, J. M., Natsuaki, M. N., . . . Thapar, A. (2013). Biological and rearing mother influences on child ADHD symptoms: Revisiting the developmental interface between nature and nurture. *Journal of Child Psychology and Psychiatry, and Allied Disciplines*, *54*(10), 1038–1046. doi:10.1111/ jcpp.12100

Herbert, S. D., Harvey, E. A., Roberts, J. L., Wichowski, K., & Lugo-Candelas, C. I. (2013). A randomized controlled trial of a parent training and emotion socialization program for families of hyperactive preschool-aged children. *Behavior Therapy*, *44*(2), 302–316. doi:10.1016/j.beth.2012.10.004

Ingoldsby, E. M. (2010). Review of interventions to improve family engagement and retention in parent and child mental health programs. *Journal of Child and Family Studies*, *19*(5), 629–645. doi:10.1007/ s10826-009-9350-2

Iznardo, M., Rogers, M. A., Volpe, R. J., Labelle, P. R., & Robaey, P. (2017). The effectiveness of daily behavior report cards for children with ADHD: A meta-analysis. *Journal of Attention Disorders*. doi:10.1177/ 1087054717734646

Jacobsen, E. (1929). *Progressive relaxation*. Chicago, IL: University of Chicago Press.

Jensen, P. S., Hinshaw, S. P., Kraemer, H. C., Lenora, N., Newcorn, J. H., Abikoff, H. B., . . . Elliott, G. R. (2001). ADHD comorbidity findings from the MTA study: Comparing comorbid subgroups. *Journal of the American Academy of Child & Adolescent Psychiatry, 40*(2), 147–158. doi:10.1097/00004583-200102000-00009

Johnston, C., & Chronis-Tuscano, A. (2014). Families and ADHD. In R. A. Barkley (Ed.), *Attention-deficit hyperactivity disorder: A handbook for diagnosis and treatment* (4th ed., pp. 191–209). New York: Guilford.

Johnston, C., Mash, E. J., Miller, N., & Ninowski, J. E. (2012). Parenting in adults with attention-deficit/hyperactivity disorder (ADHD). *Clinical Psychology Review, 32*(4), 215–228. doi:10.1016/j.cpr.2012.01.007

Kabat-Zinn, J. (1994). *Wherever you go, there you are: Mindfulness meditation in everyday life.* New York: Hyperion.

Lafrance, A., & Miller, A. P. (2020). *What to say to kids when nothing seems to work: A practical guide for parents and caregivers.* New York: Routledge.

Lafrance, A., Henderson, K. A., & Mayman, S. (2020). *Emotion-focused family therapy: A transdiagnostic model for caregiver-focused interventions.* Washington, DC: American Psychological Association. doi:10.1037/0000166-000

Lee, S. S., Chronis-Tuscano, A., Keenan, K., Pelham, W. E., Loney, J., Van Hulle, C. A., . . . Lahey, B. B. (2008). Association of maternal dopamine transporter genotype with negative parenting: Evidence for gene x environment interaction with child disruptive behavior. *Molecular Psychiatry, 15*, 548–558. doi:10.1038/mp.2008.102

Lejuez, C. W., Hopko, D. R., & Hopko, S. D. (2001). A brief behavioral activation treatment for depression: Treatment manual. *Behavior Modification, 25*(2), 255–286. doi:10.1177/0145445501252005

Lewinsohn, P. M., Munoz, R. F., Youngren, M. A., & Zeiss, A. M. (1986). *Control your depression.* New York: Simon and Schuster.

Linehan, M. M. (1993). *Skills training manual for treating borderline personality disorder.* New York: Guilford.

Linehan, M. M. (2014). *DBT skills training manual* (2nd ed.). New York: Guilford.

Luby, J. L., Barch, D. M., Whalen, D., Tillman, R., & Freedland, K. E. (2018). A randomized controlled trial of parent-child psychotherapy targeting emotion development for early childhood depression. *American Journal of Psychiatry, 175*(11), 1102–1110. doi:10.1176/appi.ajp.2018.18030321

Luman, M., Tripp, G., & Scheres, A. (2010). Identifying the neurobiology of altered reinforcement sensitivity in ADHD: A review and research agenda. *Neuroscience and Biobehavioral Reviews, 34*(5), 744–754. doi:10.1016/j.neubiorev.2009.11.021

Macphee, F. L., Merrill, B. M., Altszuler, A. R., Ramos, M. C., Gnagy, E. M., Greiner, A. R., . . . Pelham, W. E. (2019). The effect of weighted vests and stability balls with and without psychostimulant medication on classroom outcomes for children with ADHD. *School Psychology Review*, *48*(3), 276–289. doi:10.17105/SPR-2017-0151.V48-3

Mazursky-Horowitz, H., Felton, J. W., MacPherson, L., Ehrlich, K. B., Cassidy, J., Lejuez, C. W., & Chronis-Tuscano, A. (2015). Maternal emotion regulation mediates the association between adult attention-deficit/hyperactivity disorder symptoms and parenting. *Journal of Abnormal Child Psychology*, *43*(1), 121–131. doi:10.1007/s10802-014-9894-5

Mazursky-Horowitz, H., Thomas, S. R., Woods, K. E., Chrabaszcz, J. S., Deater-Deckard, K., & Chronis-Tuscano, A. (2018). Maternal executive functioning and scaffolding in families of children with and without parent-reported ADHD. *Journal of Abnormal Child Psychology*, *46*(3), 463–475. doi:10.1007/s10802-017-0289-2

Miller, L. L., Gustafsson, H. C., Tipsord, J., Song, M., Nousen, E., Dieckmann, N., & Nigg, J. T. (2018). Is the association of ADHD with socio-economic disadvantage explained by child comorbid externalizing problems or parent ADHD?. *Journal of Abnormal Child Psychology*, *46*(5), 951–963.

Miller, N. V., Degnan, K. A., Hane, A. A., Fox, N. A., & Chronis-Tuscano, A. (2019). Infant temperament reactivity and early maternal caregiving: Independent and interactive links to later childhood attention-deficit/hyperactivity disorder symptoms. *Journal of Child Psychology and Psychiatry*, *60*(1), 43–53. doi:10.1111/jcpp.12934

Miller, N. V., Hane, A. A., Degnan, K. A., Fox, N. A., & Chronis-Tuscano, A. (2019). Investigation of a developmental pathway from infant anger reactivity to childhood inhibitory control and ADHD symptoms: Interactive effects of early maternal caregiving. *Journal of Child Psychology and Psychiatry*, *60*(7), 762–772. doi:10.1111/jcpp.13047

Miller, W. R., & Rollnick, S. (2012). *Motivational interviewing: Helping people change* (3rd ed.). New York: Guilford.

Molina, B. S. G., Pelham Jr., W. E., Cheong, J., Marshal, M. P., Gnagy, E. M., & Curran, P. J. (2012). Childhood attention-deficit/hyperactivity disorder (ADHD) and growth in adolescent alcohol use: The roles of functional impairments, ADHD symptom persistence, and parental knowledge. *Journal of Abnormal Psychology*, *121*(4), 922–935. doi:10.1037/a0028260

Musick, K., & Meier, A. (2012). Assessing causality and persistence in associations between family dinners and adolescent well-being. *Journal of Marriage and Family*, *74*(3), 476–493. doi:10.1111/j.1741-3737.2012.00973.x

Nigg, J. T. (2017). *Getting ahead of ADHD: What next-generation science says about treatments that work—and how you can make them work for your child*. New York: Guilford.

Nigg, J. T., & Casey, B. J. (2005). An integrative theory of attention-deficit/hyperactivity disorder based on the cognitive and affective neurosciences. *Development and Psychopathology, 17*(3), 785–806. doi:10.1017/S0954579405050376

Nock, M. K., & Kazdin, A. E. (2005). Randomized controlled trial of a brief intervention for increasing participation in parent management training. *Journal of Consulting and Clinical Psychology, 73*(5), 872–879. doi:10.1037/0022-006X.73.5.872

Oddo, L. E., Felton, J. W., Meinzer, M. C., Mazursky-Horowitz, H., Lejuez, C. W., & Chronis-Tuscano, A. (2019). Trajectories of depressive symptoms in adolescence: The interplay of maternal emotion regulation difficulties and youth ADHD symptomatology. *Journal of Attention Disorders*. doi:10.1177/1087054719864660

Oddo, L. E., Miller, N. V., Felton, J. W., Cassidy, J., Lejuez, C. W., & Chronis-Tuscano, A. (in press). Maternal emotion dysregulation predicts parenting and adolescent emotion lability: Conditional effects of youth ADHD symptoms.

Pemberton, R., & Tyszkiewicz, M. D. F. (2016). Factors contributing to depressive mood states in everyday life: A systematic review. *Journal of Affective Disorders, 200*, 103–110. doi:10.1016/j.jad.2016.04.023

Persons, J. B. (1989). *Cognitive therapy in practice: A case formulation approach*. New York: Norton.

Pfiffner, L. J. (2011). *All about ADHD: The complete practical guide for classroom teachers*. New York: Scholastic.

Pyle, K., & Fabiano, G. A. (2017). Daily report card intervention and attention deficit hyperactivity disorder: A meta-analysis of single-case studies. *Exceptional Children, 83*(4), 378–395. doi:10.1177/0014402917706370

Reitman, D., & McMahon, R. J. (2013). Constance "Connie" Hanf (1917–2002): The mentor and the model. *Cognitive and Behavioral Practice, 20*(1), 106–116. doi:10.1016/j.cbpra.2012.02.005

Roberts, M. W., McMahon, R. J., Forehand, R., & Humphreys, L. (1978). The effect of parental instruction-giving on child compliance. *Behavior Therapy, 9*(5), 793–798. doi:10.1016/S0005-7894(78)80009-4

Sanders, M. R., Markie-Dadds, C., Tully, L. A., & Bor, W. (2000). The triple-p positive parenting program: A comparison of enhanced, standard, and self-directed behavioral family intervention for parents of children with early-onset conduct problems. *Journal of Consulting and Clinical Psychology, 68*(4), 624–640. doi:10.1037OT022-006X.68A624

Sanders, M. R., & McFarland, M. (2000). Treatment of depressed mothers with disruptive children: A controlled evaluation of cognitive behavioral family intervention. *Behavior Therapy, 31*, 89–112. doi:10.1016/S0005-7894(00)80006-4

Scott, S., & Dadds, M. R. (2009). Practitioner review: When parent training doesn't work: Theory-driven clinical strategies. *Journal of Child Psychology and Psychiatry, 50*(12), 1441–1450. doi:10.1111/j.1469-7610.2009.02161.x

Seymour, K. E., Chronis-Tuscano, A., Halldorsdottir, T., Stupica, B., Owens, K., & Sacks, T. (2012). Emotion regulation mediates the relationship between ADHD and depressive symptoms in youth. *Journal of Abnormal Child Psychology, 40*(4), 595–606. doi:10.1007/s10802-011-9593-4

Seymour, K. E., Chronis-Tuscano, A., Iwamoto, D. K., Kurdziel, G., & MacPherson, L. (2014). Emotion regulation mediates the association between ADHD and depressive symptoms in a community sample of youth. *Journal of Abnormal Child Psychology, 42*(4), 611–621. doi:10.1007/s10802-013-9799-8

Skinner, B. F. (1963). Operant behavior. *American Psychologist, 18*(8), 503. doi:10.1037/h0045185

Sonuga-Barke, E. J. (2002). Psychological heterogeneity in AD/HD: A dual pathway model of behaviour and cognition. *Behavioural Brain Research, 130*(1–2), 29–36. doi:https://doi.org/10.1016/s0166-4328(01)00432-6

Webster-Stratton, C. (1990). Enhancing the effectiveness of self-administered videotape parent training for families with conduct-problem children. *Journal of Abnormal Child Psychology, 18*(5), 479–492. doi:10.1007/bf00911103

Weisz, J. R. (2004). *Psychotherapy for children and adolescents: Evidence-based treatments and case examples.* Cambridge: Cambridge University Press.

Weisz, J. R., Chorpita, B. F., Frye, A., Ng, M. Y., Lau, N., Bearman, S. K., . . . Hoagwood, K. E. (2011). Youth top problems: Using idiographic, consumer-guided assessment to identify treatment needs and to track change during psychotherapy. *Journal of Consulting and Clinical Psychology, 79*(3), 369–380. doi:10.1037/a0023307